CW00758710

MENSTRUAL MYTH

The Case of the Hormo

Sally King

P

First published in Great Britain in 2025 by

Policy Press, an imprint of
Bristol University Press
University of Bristol
1–9 Old Park Hill
Bristol
BS2 8BB
UK
t: +44 (0)117 374 6645
e: bup-info@bristol.ac.uk

Details of international sales and distribution partners are available at policy.bristoluniversitypress.co.uk

British Library Cataloguing in Publication Data
A catalogue record for this book is available from the British Library

ISBN 978-1-4473-7162-5 hardcover
ISBN 978-1-4473-7163-2 paperback
ISBN 978-1-4473-7164-9 ePub
ISBN 978-1-4473-7165-6 ePdf

Cover design: Nicky Borowiec
Front cover image: AdobeStock/beast01
Bristol University Press and Policy Press use environmentally responsible print partners.
Printed and bound in Great Britain by CPI Group (UK) Ltd, Croydon, CR0 4YY

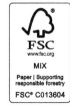

FSC
www.fsc.org
MIX
Paper | Supporting
responsible forestry
FSC® C013604

For all those whose pain has been doubted.

Contents

List of figures, tables and boxes   vii
List of abbreviations   ix
Glossary   x
Acknowledgements   xiii
Trigger warnings   xiv

Introduction   **1**
    Why this book?   1
    Why now?   3
    Why me?   5
    What's in the book?   6

PART I   **Menstrual myth making**   **9**
1   **The reduction and mystification of the menstrual cycle**   **11**
    What we should have been taught at (med) school but weren't   11
    Why we have periods (hold on to your hats!)   13
    Menstrual physiology beyond hormones   20
2   **How did we get here?**   **26**
    Female-prevalent symptoms throughout the history of medicine   26
    Key political and philosophical influences on female hysteria   29
    From hysterical to hormonal: the emergence of biomedical PMS   32
    The emergence of critical perspectives on PMS   36

PART II **Where are we now? PMS (Premenstrual Syndrome)**   **45**
3   **What counts as a premenstrual symptom?**   **47**
    Biopsychosocial factors in PMS   48
    Comparing discourses to identify commonalities, differences   52
    and omissions
    Conducting Critical Realist Discourse Analysis   55
4   **Mind over matter: the psychologisation of premenstrual changes**   **64**
    The expert prioritisation of emotional distress   64
    Premenstrual changes as 'all in her mind'   67
    Much ado about PMDD   73
    Chapter summary   78
5   **Snatch-22: premenstrual changes as simultaneously**   **82**
    'normal' and debilitating
    The medicalisation of typically mild premenstrual changes   82
    The minimisation of debilitating premenstrual symptoms   89
    Constructing the 'snatch-22' paradox   95
    Chapter summary   99

6	**The curse: femininity as debility**	**104**
	Blaming the female sex (hormones)	104
	Gendered perspectives, symptoms and treatments	108
	Exaggerating the premenstrual problem	114
	Chapter summary	120
7	**Black box: the unknown/mysterious female reproductive body**	**124**
	Ignorance is not bliss	124
	The reduction and mystification of the menstrual cycle	130
	Disciplinary dilemmas and other practical problems	136
	Chapter summary	141
8	**Conclusion and call to action**	**145**
	Bad science, but good intentions?	145
	So what? Key implications	155
	Chapter summary	158
	Call to action!	160

Appendix A: The reduction of menstrual physiology in (medical) education	165
Appendix B: Participant background survey	167
Appendix C: Interview question lists	169
Appendix D: Transcription notation	173
Appendix E: Discursive device notation	174
Appendix F: Discourse coding tree	176
Appendix G: The influence of three key gender myths on the participant group discourses	180
Notes	182
References	194
Index	217

List of figures, tables and boxes

Figures

1.1	A typical depiction of the menstrual cycle	12
1.2	The four genetic lineages of the 19 known menstruating mammals	15
2.1	Publications on premenstrual disorders per year, 1950–2018	35
2.2	Popular media images of the hysterical/hormonal female	38
2.3	PMS as gender myth: Hilary Clinton depicted as pathologically emotional due to PMS during her party leadership campaign in 2007 (when she was 60 years old!)	41
2.4	PMS as gender myth: 'Mother Nature' depicted as hysterical and subject to PMS (also despite being post-reproductive age in appearance), published in 2011	41
4.1	Top ten responses to 'PMS is considered by some to be a controversial diagnosis, what is your understanding of why this might be?'	69
4.2	The psychologisation of premenstrual changes and reproduction of the 'all in the mind' gender myth	80
5.1	Premenstrual changes as simultaneously 'normal' and debilitating	102
6.1	Average biomedical and patient PMS (and PMDD) population prevalence estimates, compared to robust prospective population data	119
6.2	Positioning the female (reproductive) body as pathological	122
7.1	Diagram depicting the PMS biomedical experts' reduction of the menstrual cycle to 'fluctuations in sex hormones' only	134
7.2	The unknown/mysterious female reproductive body	143
8.1	The three societal gender myths reflected in the four main discursive themes inductively derived from the interview data	148

Tables

2.1	Cases of Premenstrual Tension	33
2.2	A–D of the diagnostic criteria for PMDD in DSM V	36
2.3	The top ten countries publishing PMS/PMDD studies, 1945–2018	39
3.1	Participant characteristics and information	54
3.2	The top ten metaphors used to describe premenstrual experiences and their relative usage by the expert and patient participants	59

3.3	The selection criteria for, and limitations of, the four datasets used to compare with the participant descriptions of PMS	60
4.1	What are the most common premenstrual symptoms? Average number and type of symptoms mentioned by participant group	67
5.1	The inclusion of typically mild non-pathological changes in the current (DSM V) diagnostic criteria for PMDD	83
5.2	The medicalisation of certain premenstrual symptoms listed in order of usage frequency by group and compared to data derived from Dennerstein et al (2011)	88
5.3	Have you ever consulted a doctor about your premenstrual symptoms? Patient data disclosed during interviews	92
5.4	The minimisation of certain premenstrual symptoms listed in order of usage frequency by group and compared to data derived from Dennerstein et al (2011)	94
5.5	The biomedical labelling of, and clinical specialism responsible for, the top 20 most common premenstrual changes	100
6.1	Additional and overemphasised symptoms mentioned by the experts and patients, in comparison with population data derived from Dennerstein et al (2011)	111
6.2	The 17 core symptoms described by the participant groups and included in the DSM criteria for PMDD	115
7.1	Results of an NVivo text frequency query regarding 'dirty/toxic' metaphors used to describe premenstrual experiences	126
7.2	Results of NVivo text frequency queries regarding terms relating to healthy (pre)menstrual physiology	132
8.1	Comparison of the claims made in participant group descriptions of premenstrual symptoms versus the available population data	147
8.2	The key enabling and constraining discursive mechanisms and extra-discursive factors affecting participant group descriptions of PMS	152
8.3	The demonstrated intentions of the five discursive mechanisms and extra-discursive factors explicitly discussed by the participants	154

Boxes

1.1	The reduction and mystification of the menstrual cycle: why this matters	23
2.1	From hysterical to hormonal: why this matters	42
3.1	What counts as a premenstrual symptom? Why this matters	62
4.1	Mind over matter: why this matters	80
5.1	Snatch-22: why this matters	102
6.1	The curse: why this matters	122
7.1	Black box: why this matters	144
8.1	Moving forward in women's health: you!	164

List of abbreviations

CRDA	Critical Realist Discourse Analysis
DA	Discourse Analysis
DP	Discursive Psychology
DSM	Diagnostic and Statistical Manual of Mental Disorders
GP	General Practitioner
IBS	irritable bowel syndrome
LLPDD	Late Luteal Phase Dysphoric Disorder
PMDD	Premenstrual Dysphoric Disorder
PME	premenstrual exacerbation
PMS	Premenstrual Syndrome
PMT	Premenstrual Tension
RCOG	Royal College of Obstetricians and Gynaecologists (UK)
SD	spontaneous decidualisation

Glossary

Decidualisation   The thickening of the womb lining in preparation for pregnancy

Dysmenorrhea   Painful (and perhaps heavy) menstruation/periods

Epidemiology   The study of population health or illness characteristics

Follicular (phase)   The first half of an average ovarian cycle, starting at menstruation and continuing until ovulation, when an egg (follicle) is released from the ovary

Late Luteal Phase Dysphoric Disorder   The diagnostic precursor to the psychiatric disorder now known as PMDD

Luteal (phase)   The second half of an average ovarian cycle, starting at ovulation and ending at the start of menstruation

Menstruation (periods)   The regular and healthy process by which the lining and contents of the womb are shed from the body to protect females of reproductive age from potentially dangerous or inviable pregnancies

Mixed methods   Research conducted using a combination of qualitative and quantitative methods and/or data

Oestrus   Conspicuous ovulation or fertile phases in most but not all mammals. Humans conceal ovulation and we are typically unaware of our fertility

Ovulation   The physiological process by which a mammalian egg (ovule) is released from the ovary, initiating the fertile phase in which heterosexual copulation may result in pregnancy

Premenstrual Dysphoric Disorder   Severe emotional distress experienced only in the luteal phase of the menstrual cycle. Diagnosis is based on the meeting of certain criteria outlined in the DSM

Premenstrual exacerbation	The triggering or worsening of an underlying health issue at certain times in the menstrual cycle (typically from ovulation up to and including menstruation)
Premenstrual Syndrome	Any cyclical changes that significantly impair an individual. Typically occurring a week to ten days before, and perhaps also during the first couple of days of menstruation
Premenstrual Tension	The precursor diagnostic label to PMS, but with a specific focus on emotional distress
Positivist/Realist	The 17th-century philosophical idea that *all* of reality can be objectively and empirically observed, understood, and measured by humans. This (contested) theory underpins many of the methodologies promoted within Western medicine
Qualitative (research methods or data)	A process of inquiry that seeks to gain an in-depth understanding of social phenomena. It enables 'why' and 'how' questions to be answered (which quantitative inquiry alone cannot)
Quantitative (research methods or data)	A process of inquiry that seeks to gain a generalisable understanding of social phenomena. It enables 'what' questions to be answered (which qualitative inquiry alone cannot)
Social constructionist	An interpretivist theory of knowledge. Given that knowledge of all things is always mediated by human culture and language, some perceived 'social facts' may actually reproduce human cultural beliefs and values rather than describe a 'real' entity or experience
Spontaneous decidualisation	Automatic thickening of the womb lining (in response to rising progesterone levels) that triggers regular periods in a tiny minority of mammals, regardless of ovulation, copulation, conception or pregnancy status

Stereotype   A popular and highly recognisable depiction of a population group, typically negative, and serving to justify discriminatory beliefs and practices

Symptom   In this study context, any embodied experience that causes discomfort or distress to an extent that prevents typical physical or social activities

Acknowledgements

This research would not have been possible without funding provided by the Economic and Social Research Council (grant numbers: 1916672, ES/Y007816/1) and the Sociological Review Fellowship. Thanks to King's College London and Keele University for supporting my research, given that no university (in the world!) currently teaches healthy menstrual physiology. Thanks especially to my Sociological Review mentors and colleagues, and the Jonas lab at King's – it was so nice to feel welcome, even if my work is a little different.

Thanks so much to my family and friends who have kept me going over the past decade. Your cuddles, chats, walks, swims, invites to coffee, lunch, pints and Zoom calls were most appreciated. Plus, if it wasn't for an unexpected inheritance from Aunty Joan and the distinct feeling that she would want me to 'do something' with it, I couldn't have got into menstrual health research in the first place.

Thanks to the Society for Menstrual Cycle Research for creating one of the kindest and most welcoming professional networks possible. Thanks also to my friends and colleagues from the ever-growing UK and global menstrual health and rights movement, it's often a difficult and risky road to take, but at least we are not alone.

Most of all, I'd like to thank my study participants, your experiences and words literally made this book. I've done my best to represent your contributions as fairly and transparently as possible and I really hope that the findings are of value to you.

Finally, Mammy, you once said something that really stuck with me: 'Take a look around! See what needs doing and just do it!' It turns out that this is pretty solid advice for a researcher… Thanks.

Trigger warnings

This book discusses the following potentially distressing topics: menstrual stigma; sexism; racism; spontaneous (non-medical) abortion; miscarriage; maternal mortality; suicide; and gender-based violence.

Introduction

For the past several years, I have been terrified that something would happen to me or for some other reason I wouldn't be able to share these research findings. The idea that decades, even centuries, from now people might *still* be dismissing and diminishing women's accounts of pain and distress, simply due to the myth of the 'hysterical/hormonal female' has been a highly motivating, but also anxiety-inducing fear. I am so happy and *relieved* to have made it this far. Now the burden of knowledge will be shared with everyone who reads this book!

Why this book?

One day, I will write an accessible learning resource, full of wonderful pictures and fun facts, describing everything we should all be taught about our reproductive bodies. But this book had to come first.

You see, I am not the first person to point out inconsistencies and omissions in medical discourses, especially regarding female (reproductive) health. The famous 17th-century physician, Thomas Willis, openly criticised his colleagues who blamed the womb/hysteria for any unexplained symptoms in their female patients (quoted at length in Chapter 2).[1] Mary Putnam Jacobi, one of the first women to (be allowed to) qualify as a doctor in the 19th century, was forced to prove that periods did not actually make girls and women 'unsuited' to education and the professions.[2] In the early 1930s, Karen Horney critiqued the first formal description of 'Premenstrual Tension', realising immediately how its gynaecological categorisation would reinforce sexist beliefs about the psychological weakness of 'all women'.[3] In 1949, Simone de Beauvoir revealed the role of the hysterical female trope in maintaining the inferior political status of women.[4] Then, more recently, numerous feminist scholars have drawn attention to the political value of medicalising/pathologising the menstrual cycle, in particular. Perhaps most notably, Emily Martin,[5] Anne Walker,[6] Sophie Laws,[7] Paula Caplan,[8] Anne Figert,[9] Joan Chrisler,[10] Jane Ussher,[11] Janette Perz[12] and Robyn Stein DeLuca.[13]

The problem is that this more recent critical literature (outlined in detail in Chapter 2) is often wrongly interpreted by clinicians, biomedical researchers and the public as positioning cyclic symptoms as somehow 'unreal'. As a result, the work of these feminist scholars is dismissed (often without even being read) by those who need to engage with it the most. Of course, if you stop and think for a moment, this interpretation doesn't make much sense. Why would a feminist dismiss or deny women's experiences? The point they are trying to make is that the application of *medical* labels to the *healthy* changes experienced by most people who menstruate is inappropriate. What is more, by pathologising the menstrual cycle, sexist beliefs about the 'natural' biological inferiority of women are perpetuated. The fact that a minority of individuals do experience cyclic symptoms is *not* denied, these are instead attributed to underlying conditions or distress associated with having periods, a highly stigmatised and often painful experience.

My worry, then, is that regardless of the quality of my work, and the data upon which it is based, I too might struggle to be believed by others. An ironic situation faced by any woman trying to debunk the myth of the hysterical female, I guess! As a result, this academic book is a chance to carefully and transparently share my methods, data, findings and conclusions, to encourage you, the reader, to make up your own mind about the validity of these claims. This book is entirely open to critical scrutiny, you can even access the original (anonymised) interview data.[14]

Unfortunately, because of this 'full transparency' approach, less specialist readers may find some chapters a little challenging to read. The good news is that each chapter has a summary or 'why this matters' section at the end, which contains the main takeaway points. This is basically all you really need to know, and the rest of the chapter simply provides the material required to back up these findings. This way I hope to have made the book as accessible as possible, while providing all the information needed to make an informed interpretation of its arguments.

I have also tried to integrate the various, typically separate, strands of existing PMS (Premenstrual Syndrome) research and data. For too long, critical perspectives have been assumed to be 'at odds' with the biomedical literature, when it is perfectly possible to treat them as complementary discourses. Distinguishing healthy pre/menstrual changes from pathological cyclical symptoms is not as difficult as the literature might have you believe. Especially once you realise that cyclical symptoms are not merely a 'more severe version' of healthy menstrual physiology (discussed in Chapters 1, 4 and 5). Integrating critical and biomedical data is something I do automatically, as a medical sociologist who reads 'both sides' of the story, plus everything else I can get my hands on from historical, epidemiological and physiological sources too. In fact, I avoid applying a feminist methodology or approach in my own research (outlined in Chapter 3), partly to reassure clinicians and biomedical colleagues that I am not taking any particular side.

My drive to integrate critical with biomedical perspectives on PMS stems from a frustration at the needless limitations affecting both traditions. Critical scholars have historically avoided biological explanations for women's experiences, perhaps in fear of giving credence to sexist 'essentialist' beliefs (the idea that gender inequalities are based on biology rather than power relations). I argue, however, that it is important to directly engage with biological data, to expose and critique any (unintentional) biases in its interpretation (Chapters 1, 7 and 8). Similarly, most biomedical PMS experts have failed to engage with the available critical research regarding external (non-biological) factors in cyclical symptoms (Chapters 2 and 3). This is even more inexplicable given that most of us are all too aware of the impact life stressors can have on our health. This is not new or controversial science. Therefore, the book aims to provide an alternative (evidence-based and holistic) explanation for the female prevalence of certain symptoms, without reinforcing any gender norms.

Alas, our collective ignorance of healthy menstrual physiology is so profound that even when well-meaning activists, researchers and health professionals try to do something about this gap in our education, they often end up reproducing the very same myths and misconceptions that have limited our knowledge for centuries. Every period education book I've ever read implies or directly states that menstruation 'helps prepare for' pregnancy, and that typical cyclical changes are 'hormonal' in origin (both myths are debunked in Chapter 1). Even Dr Jen Gunter, a famously straight-talking feminist gynaecologist, positions periods as 'optimizing pregnancy outcomes' and attributes premenstrual changes to 'hormonal fluctuations'.[15] What hope do the rest of us have when even gynaecologists are not adequately taught about healthy menstrual physiology?[16] Where ignorance reigns, societal myths quickly fill the gaps. Hence, menstrual health literacy becomes an urgent and crucial global intervention for improving gender equality, as well as our health and wellbeing.

Why now?

I'm sure to some readers it might seem like menstrual and menopausal health is all over the newspapers, television and social media these days. The last few years have certainly seen an increase in the visibility of menstrual health issues but, unfortunately, no real improvement in menstrual or menopausal health literacy or effective treatments for related conditions. Much of this recent content comes from activists, journalists, celebrities and grassroots patient support groups desperate to share more accessible and trustworthy information on these topics.[17] The problem is that we are not currently taught enough about healthy menstrual physiology (or how to spot sexist tropes) to create evidence-based resources and not (however unintentionally) reproduce societal myths.

For instance, when we talk about period poverty, the focus is typically 'periods as a reason why some girls are missing school'.[18] This, unfortunately, frames the healthy female reproductive body as the problem rather than the government policies that directly contribute to increasing poverty, or the fact that most schools (and workplaces) are still not fit for people who menstruate, or the huge profit margins gained from the sale of expensive disposable period products. In fact, period poverty media coverage often provides free marketing for the very companies that help create the problem in the first place. Similarly, a recent UK campaign to abolish the 'tampon tax' has unintentionally boosted the profits of disposable product manufacturers by about £15 million per year, without reducing the cost of products for consumers.[19] As Chris Bobel also concluded in relation to the 'menstrual hygiene' movement within the international development sector, due to our collective ignorance, blaming the healthy menstruating body appears to be a more familiar narrative groove for us, than one that dares challenge political inequalities and profiteering companies.[20]

Then we have the trending topic of 'menstrual/menopause leave', which has even supposedly feminist groups lobbying for days (even months) off school and paid employment, for 'all' women and girls. Again, the healthy female reproductive body is positioned as the problem rather than inadequate work environments, toxic cultures that penalise rest breaks or the uptake of sick leave (when needed), global menstrual/menopausal health illiteracy, and the tendency of medicine to pathologise healthy reproductive processes while simultaneously minimising severe cyclic or menopausal symptoms (discussed in Chapters 2 and 5). While we do need workplace interventions, these should be educational initiatives of benefit to all employees, not a sex-specific sick leave.[21] Implying that periods or the menopause are debilitating for most women is simply not true and reproduces dangerous discriminatory beliefs. Plus, the minority of people experiencing severe cyclic or menopausal symptoms require support, and ideally effective treatment, for their underlying conditions. They do not deserve to be excluded from school or the workplace and made to suffer in silence alone at home.[22]

There's also been recent media coverage regarding the myth of the 'hysterical female' in patient accounts of poor clinical practices and outcomes. The ongoing dismissal of painful complications relating to vaginal mesh implants,[23] the horrific case of the Yale fertility clinic that ignored the cries of over 200 women undergoing excruciating egg-retrieval surgery without anaesthetic,[24] unnecessary delays of several years in the diagnosis of endometriosis,[25] and gender and racial biases in the (lack of) treatment of women's pain.[26] While many patients allude to the myth of the 'hysterical female' in their accounts of poor treatment, very little attention has been paid to how this myth persists within the medical encounter. I doubt that many clinicians truly believe that women are somehow biologically prone to inventing, exaggerating or imagining painful symptoms – and yet, time after time, this is how we are ultimately treated. To my mind, the gap in our collective knowledge regarding our reproductive bodies enables this myth to thrive. Without any better explanation, we unconsciously resort to accessible folk tales.

Given that 'hysteria' is a label also applied to racialised, colonised and otherwise marginalised populations (discussed in Chapters 2 and 4), I am pleased to see that recent work regarding institutional racial and colonial biases is already paving the way for changes in medical training. In particular, Malone Mukwende's identification of the lack of representation of patients with darker skin tones in textbook depictions of a range of health conditions. Mukwende's co-authored *Mind the Gap* handbook aims to bridge this current gap in training,[27] but there has also been widespread public interest and support for the inclusion of more representative imagery within core medical textbooks and the National Health Service website.[28] Similarly, Anabel Sowemimo's book, *Divided: Racism, Medicine and Why We Need to Decolonise Healthcare*, seems to have ignited some much-needed institutional interest from the likes of the *British Medical Journal*, and others, in teaching medical students and clinicians about some of the racial, colonial, gendered and class biases inherent within their training.[29]

In short, it is a pretty good time to be sharing this research. By filling you in on what has been absent from your education so far and illustrating the way in which this omission shapes our descriptions and interpretations of female-prevalent symptoms, together we might be able to banish the myth of the hysterical/hormonal female once and for all.

Why me?

Given the highly contested nature of this topic, it is crucial that I share something of my personal experiences and perspectives, to enable a more informed reading of the book.

I first became interested in researching this topic in 2012, after experiencing progressively worsening nausea and vomiting symptoms for a couple of years. After several inconclusive blood tests and gastrointestinal examinations, my symptoms were eventually diagnosed as 'anxiety', despite the fact I was not really experiencing any. Rather than accepting this diagnosis and the subsequent prescription for anti-anxiety medication (plus 'mood stabilisers' due to a familial rather than personal history of bipolar disorder), I decided to keep a record of my symptoms in case there was some sort of food or lifestyle trigger. Within three months, I had identified a pattern relating to the menstrual cycle, and within a year, I had substantially alleviated my symptoms through some simple lifestyle changes.

At the time, I was a professional researcher designing and conducting mixed-method evaluations of human rights campaigns, policies and interventions – typically with a focus on gender equality. I had a master's degree in (qualitative and quantitative) research methods, an undergraduate degree in anthropology and an active interest in the natural sciences, which I had studied up to sixth form (age 18) and then again in several adult education courses. As a result, I was (by chance) somewhat well placed to notice the way in which social norms seemed to prevent doctors and patients from discussing or considering the role of the menstrual cycle in female ill-health, unless done so through 'psychological' or 'psychiatric' diagnostic labels and explanations.

I began to research menstrual health in my spare time, then one day per week, until eventually I decided to work on it full time (unfunded). The Menstrual Matters website was launched in early 2016.[30] The website provides evidence-based information about how to identify and manage common premenstrual changes and cyclical health issues, and shares educational blogs about menstrual physiology, the history of medicine, and the ways in which menstrual taboos relate to discriminatory beliefs and practices. The website currently attracts around 60,000 users per month, and its crowd science 'symptom checker' application has compiled anonymised cyclical symptom data from over 2,000 individuals.

As a result of writing several blogs on this topic, I was first asked to present my work on 'PMS and the myth of the irrational female' at the 2016 Society for Menstrual Cycle Research conference in Atlanta. This eventually became a chapter in the *Palgrave Handbook of Critical Menstruation Studies*.[31] It was this preliminary research (and the need to establish greater academic credibility in the field) that prompted me to undertake a PhD in medical sociology. I completed my doctoral research in 2022, and this book is directly based on that study.

What's in the book?

The book is split into two parts. The first part provides the reader with some useful background information about the menstrual cycle (beyond hormones) and the contested history of medicine regarding female prevalent and cyclical symptoms. The second part uses the example of PMS to illustrate the way in which societal myths, such as the hysterical/hormonal female, continue to influence medical, critical and popular descriptions of women's health.

Chapter 1 will teach you some of things we should have been taught at school but weren't. You may find some of these things shocking because they fundamentally challenge pervasive beliefs about the female body. I suggest you try to keep calm and read the chapter in full before examining any emotional response you may experience. It is perfectly normal to feel anger, disbelief or confusion when confronted with this information. I can assure you it is all evidence-based and thoroughly peer-reviewed.

Chapter 2 explains how we got into this mess in the first place. Why are we still being taught sexist ideology rather than evidence-based information about our bodies? It turns out that an ancient medical tendency to attribute female-prevalent symptoms to 'femininity' (first the womb, now the sex hormones) continues to act as an unacknowledged metaphor within medical discourses. The chapter summarises both the biomedical and critical literatures on hysteria and PMS, to provide the historical and intellectual context to the present study.

Chapter 3 explains a bit more about the work that has already been done on the biological, social and psychological factors impacting menstrual health. I then describe the people I interviewed in my PMS study, the theory and methodology I used to gather and analyse the data, and provide some examples of how the method was applied.

The following four chapters (Chapters 4–7) take each of the main themes identified in the interview data ('mind over matter', 'snatch-22', 'the curse' and 'black box') and describe their constitutive sub-themes. Quotes from my interview participants are used to illustrate each point, either for the way in which they spoke or for what they spoke about. Remember, you are also able to access the original data, to see the original quotes in full and within their interview context.[32]

The final chapter (Chapter 8) brings everything together and summarises the main findings of this study and their key implications for science, clinical practice, society and each of us as individuals. It ends with a slightly cheesy but heartfelt call to action. Yes, it may come across as a bit preachy, but this is a rare chance to record these thoughts in writing. Again, feel free to come to your own conclusions about how we might do better in the future – I am just trying to start a much-needed conversation. I look forward to hearing your thoughts.

PART I

Menstrual myth making

1

The reduction and mystification of the menstrual cycle

My doctoral research involved interviewing nearly half of the world's leading biomedical experts on Premenstrual Syndrome (PMS). During the interview process I began to wonder why none of them were talking about menstrual physiology aside from references to 'hormones'. This was quite a shocking revelation to me because through my own research, I knew a lot more about menstrual physiology beyond its hormonal coordination. I had presumed that this was something taught to all medical students or, at the very least, those specialising in gynaecology. But I was wrong.

A subsequent analysis of 14 of the top textbooks used to train medical students found that menstrual physiology beyond its hormonal coordination is almost completely absent (Appendix A).[1] This means that no one, not even gynaecologists (other than some who later specialise in infertility research), is adequately taught about healthy menstrual physiology. This is pretty alarming! I am a seasoned researcher specialising in this topic and I had no idea about this educational omission until I reviewed these textbooks. I genuinely believed that sexist beliefs had largely been identified and stripped from school and medical textbooks following the highly influential work of Emily Martin in the 1980s.[2] Yet, what started off as a simple desire to better educate people about their bodies has become a mission to counter nearly a century of inadequate and arguably discriminatory (medical) education.

The first part of this book, therefore, is designed to help you better understand and reflect on my findings regarding expert and lay descriptions of PMS. Given that most readers will not be infertility specialists, the chapter starts with an outline of what we are typically taught at (medical) school and then, more importantly, what we are not taught. The various scientific, clinical, societal and personal implications of these omissions are then discussed.

What we should have been taught at (med) school but weren't

In many countries, children must be taught something about the menstrual cycle as part of their mandatory high school education. As a result, you should be somewhat familiar with Figure 1.1 (even if the associated facts are perhaps a little hazy)?

Figure 1.1: A typical depiction of the menstrual cycle

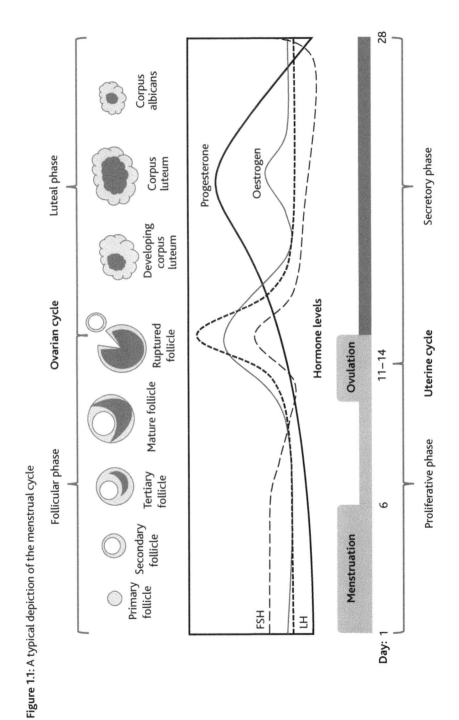

You have probably been taught about the fluctuating levels of four key reproductive hormones (follicle stimulating hormone [FSH], luteinising hormone [LH], oestrogen and progesterone) and how these changes coordinate the events occurring in an average 28-day menstrual cycle.[3]

You might also have been taught that the ovarian cycle is divided into two main phases; the follicular phase (when an egg follicle starts to develop ready to be released from an ovary) and the luteal phase (from ovulation up to the start of menstruation – when an egg pushes through the wall of an ovary and moves towards the womb).[4]

Finally, you likely learnt how the lining of the womb (endometrium) gets much thicker during the second half of the uterine cycle and then, if no pregnancy occurs, this tissue is shed from the body during menstruation (the period), after a sudden drop in progesterone.[5] If you studied a biomedical degree at university, you will have revised more or less the same content, albeit in greater molecular detail (Appendix A).[6] If you went on to specialise in gynaecology, you might have been taught about abnormal uterine changes and associated conditions, but not much more regarding healthy menstrual physiology (Appendix A).[7] In short, the hormonal coordination of ovulation and menstruation is the main, if not only, element of menstrual physiology currently taught to children, nurses, general medical practitioners and gynaecologists (unless you go on to specialise in infertility or a menstrual health condition, such as endometriosis or abnormal heavy bleeding).

What is so wrong with teaching children, research scientists and clinicians this reduced version of menstrual physiology? After all, we do not have time to learn absolutely everything about the human body. The implications will be discussed throughout this book, but for now let us begin with what is not currently covered in our menstrual education: the purpose of periods; menstrual physiology beyond hormonal fluctuations; some common cyclic changes; and why these things *really* matter.

Why we have periods (hold on to your hats!)

I often start talks and workshops with a seemingly simple question to participants: 'Why is it that humans menstruate, given that 98 per cent of mammals do not?' It certainly feels like something we should have been taught at school. Especially because half of the population will experience periods at some point in our lives. Amidst the confused and embarrassed mumbling and shaking of heads this question typically elicits, I sometimes ask an even more unsettling one: 'Why have you never asked?' We will now work through these questions together, but I would also like you to reflect on what you learn here that you were not taught at (med) school, and why you probably did not question these omissions, or what you *were* taught.

Let us start with the first question. Why *do* humans menstruate? To make things a little easier, I will provide a multiple-choice list of possible answers. Simply pick the one that you feel best fits what you have gleaned through life experience, exposure to media and any formal education:

A. To clean out the womb.
B. It is a type of natural abortion.
C. To prepare for pregnancy.
D. To protect us from danger (even death!).
E. To signal our fertility.
F. Two of these answers combined … (and which ones?).
G. All of these things.
H. We don't know.

The most common answers I hear are A, C or E (or F relating to two of these answers). Yet, the correct answer is F – options B and D. Periods are a type of natural abortion[8] and the most likely reason they evolved is to help protect us from the (potentially fatal) dangers of human pregnancy and childbirth. This is probably not what you thought. In fact, it might be the opposite to what you thought, and we will find out why shortly. However, before we go through why you might have felt strongly drawn to A, C, E or H, let us run through the rationale behind answers B and D.

The evidence base

As beautifully argued by evolutionary biologists, Emera, Romero and Wagner, over a decade ago, the regular shedding of the womb lining and everything in it most likely performs an abortive role.[9] To make their case, Emera and colleagues compared data from across the entire mammalian family tree (Figure 1.2). To begin with, periods are a surprisingly rare thing.[10] Out of over 5,000 types of placental mammals, *all* ovulate but only 84 species menstruate (approximately 1.6 per cent).[11] This select group includes us humans, our ape cousins, most old world monkeys, some new world monkeys, four species of bats, the elephant shrew and (only recently discovered) the spiny mouse.[12] Such random diversity reveals that menstruation has evolved independently at least four times along different genetic lines (Figure 1.2). This suggests that periods probably provide some form of survival advantage.[13]

Crucially, Emera and colleagues also found that menstruating mammals had other things in common (aside from regular bleeding), including a physiological process known as *spontaneous decidualisation*. In fact, it turns out that periods are a direct result of spontaneous decidualisation.[14] Spontaneous just means 'automatic' and 'decidualisation' refers to the growth and

Figure 1.2: The four genetic lineages of the 19 known menstruating mammals

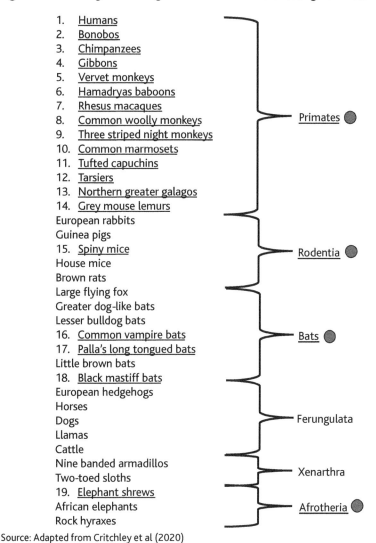

1. Humans
2. Bonobos
3. Chimpanzees
4. Gibbons
5. Vervet monkeys
6. Hamadryas baboons
7. Rhesus macaques
8. Common woolly monkeys
9. Three striped night monkeys
10. Common marmosets
11. Tufted capuchins
12. Tarsiers
13. Northern greater galagos
14. Grey mouse lemurs
European rabbits
Guinea pigs
15. Spiny mice
House mice
Brown rats
Large flying fox
Greater dog-like bats
Lesser bulldog bats
16. Common vampire bats
17. Palla's long tongued bats
Little brown bats
18. Black mastiff bats
European hedgehogs
Horses
Dogs
Llamas
Cattle
Nine banded armadillos
Two-toed sloths
19. Elephant shrews
African elephants
Rock hyraxes

Primates

Rodentia

Bats

Ferungulata

Xenarthra

Afrotheria

Source: Adapted from Critchley et al (2020)

transformation of certain cells lining the womb (often described as *thickening*) referred to as 'SD' from now on.

In 98 per cent of mammals (that is, those who do not menstruate) decidualisation of the lining of the womb *only* happens in response to hormones released by a fertilised egg as it tries to attach to it. In menstruating species, however, decidualisation happens on a regular basis, automatically.[15] This means it occurs even if we have not ovulated that month, or had sex (ever), and even if there is no egg present in the womb (fertilised or not). For us, decidualisation is automatically triggered by rising levels of progesterone, 7–10 days before the period arrives.

Emera and colleagues present two complementary theories regarding the purpose of menstruation, given that it seems to be a consequence of SD.[16] The first is that the decidualisation happens ahead of any *potential* pregnancy, to provide 'earlier and more effective protection' against dangerous placental attachments – the connecting tissue formed between the parent and foetus. Supporting this theory is the fact that menstruating species, especially humans, experience invasive placental attachments, where the life of the parent may be put at risk by the demands of the foetus. The second theory is that the process of SD enables the early detection and elimination of any fertilised eggs with genetic or other types of abnormalities (humans also have exceptionally high rates of such abnormalities).[17]

Therefore, if the placenta is too deeply or insufficiently embedded in the womb, or an abnormal fertilised egg is detected, menstruation prevents the potentially costly, even fatal, consequences of a defective or otherwise unviable pregnancy. Similarly, if no fertilised egg is present (as is the case in the vast majority of cycles) menstruation occurs because no viable pregnancy is detected.

These theories fit the available data very well. They also help to explain why such an adaptation is relevant to our species, given that humans are not very good at conceiving, maintaining a pregnancy or surviving childbirth, in comparison to most mammals. The chance of us getting pregnant per cycle – while having regular heterosexual sex without using contraception – is only one in four (25 per cent);[18] estimates for the prevalence of spontaneous abortions/miscarriages from conception to birth range from 40 per cent to 60 per cent;[19] and around the world 800 women still die *every day* due to complications relating to pregnancy and childbirth.[20]

The reason why you may find this information a bit shocking is that it runs contrary to popular belief, previous theories and even what many physiology textbooks currently imply.[21] Going through the (incorrect) options, A, C, E and H, should help you to better understand and counter some pervasive and influential gender myths that have stood in the way of evidence-based explanations of menstruation.

The myths

A. Periods clean out the womb

This is a very old and common misconception endorsed by many different populations, interest groups and philosophies. Each of the five major religions (Christianity, Islam, Hinduism, Judaism and Buddhism) have texts or present-day practices that position menstruation (and, by extension, the female body) as 'impure'.[22] Right now, in 2024, every known culture, nation and population group reacts to menstrual fluid in a very different way to other forms of blood loss. Even in supposedly feminist new age and alternative 'empowering' accounts of menstruation, the period is often portrayed as a process of *detoxification*, implying some form of impurity or pathology in the female reproductive body.

While periods can certainly stain clothes, they are not inherently dirty or dangerous. Inks, foods and blood from other parts of the body also stain clothes but have not resulted in thousands of years of prohibitive laws, social and political exclusion, and near-universal ignorance of their source or composition. For instance, it was not until 2001 that clinical researchers realised that blood only makes up around half of menstrual fluid.[23] The other half is a silky-smooth clear substance full of wonderful things such as stem cells. These cells help repair the womb lining in just five days, whereas most wounds take four to six weeks to heal.[24]

Of course, bleeding is scary because it is associated with injuries and death. Blood coming from the vaginal opening is reminiscent of childbirth; a dangerous time for humans, especially the global majority who still lack access to reproductive healthcare.[25] However, it is pretty easy to spot the difference between a healthy period and childbirth. The universal 'impurity' taboo on menstruation is, thus, not particularly well explained by its symbolic relationship with other forms of blood loss.

Periods are not a type of waste product, such as urine (wee) or faeces (poo), but, to be fair, they do leave the body from a nearby exit! However, they do not typically contain toxins, pathogens or any other harmful substances. If you have a blood-borne disease or infection, there is a tiny risk of transmission if another person comes into contact with your menstrual fluid, but the chances of this happening are extremely low. Again, the likelihood that the menstrual taboo stems from an *observable* link between periods and the transmission of illness seems highly unlikely.

Therefore, the most likely explanation for this persistent unfounded belief is widespread ignorance, which in turn enables and 'justifies' gender myths. Johnston-Robledo and Chrisler's sublime paper, 'The menstrual mark: Menstruation as social stigma', outlines such processes in detail, but, in short, by positioning menstruation (a female signifier) as physically, spiritually and morally dirty (or even 'sacred'), women are Othered from, and made inferior to, men.[26]

C. Periods help prepare for pregnancy

This is the most common answer I hear. It is not too much of a surprise, given that even specialist gynaecological physiology textbooks unhelpfully position the entire menstrual cycle (not just the ovulation part) as 'for' pregnancy.[27] But just think about it for a minute. How can the regular destruction and removal of the contents of the womb (including any fertilised eggs) *after* ovulation possibly help support a pregnancy? It cannot. This is, after all, why most successful pregnancies involve the absence of periods. However, this straightforward logical deduction has not stopped people from trying to prove otherwise.

Emera and colleagues summarise three previous hypotheses regarding the purpose of menstruation. One of these hypotheses clearly reproduces the belief that periods must somehow (despite all the evidence to the contrary) help prepare for pregnancy.[28] The idea is that the regular removal of womb lining acts as a means of 'preconditioning' the womb for the inflammatory processes (and associated risks) involved in an embryo's placental attachment. It is also claimed that periods reduce the risk of pregnancy-related (and potentially fatal) conditions such as pre-eclampsia.

Unfortunately for the researchers involved, there is little data to support these claims. As argued by Emera and colleagues, the hypothesis does not take into account that most mammals manage to conceive and give birth successfully without the need for periods. This means it does not explain why menstruation, a costly process in terms of pain and blood loss, evolved in the first place. There is also a distinct lack of experimental evidence to support the claim that periods protect against deep placental implantation (in the following reproductive cycle) or any other inflammatory health conditions.[29] Finally, I would argue that the hundreds of women still dying daily from pre-eclampsia (the third most common cause of maternal mortality),[30] a condition that does not seem to affect other menstruating species, contradicts the idea that periods confer much protection against it.[31]

If there is no compelling evidence behind the belief that periods 'help prepare for pregnancy', why does it continue to influence research and popular opinion? Again, it seems as though a gender myth has trumped the available scientific data. In this case, the idea that women and girls are *for* having and caring for children. This is another old idea used to try and justify political inequalities between men and women. Just because the female body has additional reproductive powers (pregnancy, childbirth and breast-feeding) motherhood has often been positioned as a woman's natural and main purpose and responsibility in life (as opposed to education or paid employment, for example).[32]

The idea that the female body has evolved to prioritise *our* health and wellbeing over the survival of a fertilised egg or foetus challenges this assumption, and so is rejected without adequate consideration. I cannot think of any other explanation for how generations of highly educated and well-meaning researchers and health practitioners have overlooked the fact that the removal of the womb's contents after ovulation *must* play an abortive and, thus, protective role for the parent.

E. Periods signal fertility

While it is true that someone who has regular periods is more likely to be fertile than someone who does not (due to a health issue, contraception or their age), there is no direct relationship between periods and an individual's fertility. It is perfectly possible to have regular periods yet be infertile, just as it is possible to have scant or infrequent periods and yet still produce eggs and become pregnant. Also, by the time the period arrives, any egg present would typically be unviable,[33] which makes periods a rather unhelpful signal of fertility.

In fact, humans uniquely *conceal* ovulation, which some experts in pre-eclampsia believe could be another evolutionary adaptation to help reduce the risk of death during pregnancies.[34] Indeed, we have to measure menstrual cycle length, basal body temperature, cervical position and vaginal discharge composition (or urinary hormones on a daily basis) to stand any chance of accurately charting ovulation.[35] Again, I cannot help but conclude that the 'periods indicate fertility' idea is actually down to widespread ignorance and gender norms that position women as 'for' pregnancy, childbirth and childcare.

H. We don't know why we have periods

Sure, I am willing to accept that lots of people, including doctors, believe that because they have not been taught the purpose of menstruation, that the evidence base for any one theory must be lacking. However, even if you did not previously know about the 2012 paper by Emera and colleagues, I would argue that this is a flimsy excuse. It does not take any specialist knowledge to observe that the loss of the contents of the womb after ovulation acts as an abortion. Similarly, witnessing so many people struggle to conceive, have miscarriages, get very ill or even die during pregnancy and childbirth should surely prompt us to deduce that this regular removal of the contents of the womb might play some sort of protective role? Why have we been so collectively blinkered to seeing what has been in front of our eyes for centuries (ever since we have known about sexual reproduction)?

Since there is no scientific rationale, it *must* be due to social biases or beliefs. In this instance, I argue that we are dealing with ignorance underpinned by a related gender myth: the *mysterious* female (body). Of course, the internal location of female reproductive physiology does make it relatively more mysterious than that of male bodies. However, we have now accrued over a century of reproductive health knowledge and practice, which should have enabled us to identify the likely purpose of menstruation long ago.

By positioning the female (reproductive) body as mysterious, it is possible to frame all the available data that challenge pro-natalist beliefs about it, as 'strange' rather than evidence to the contrary. The idea that we regularly experience natural abortions that have the power to terminate a pregnancy does not fit with deeply held beliefs about the designated role of women within society. Rather than questioning these inherited beliefs and gender norms, it seems easier to mystify and dismiss the credibility of challenging data, even if this goes against scientific methods (and, arguably, common sense).

Menstrual physiology beyond hormones

This section is designed to provide you with enough new knowledge to better understand and reflect on the findings discussed in the second part of this book. It is not a complete account of healthy menstrual physiology because that would require a whole book (which does not yet exist)! In fact, I am going to focus on just two key components because they are most relevant to the discussion of cyclical experiences: inflammation and iron deficiency. Before we start, though, we need to talk about hormones.

Crucially, and again contrary to popular belief, a direct *causal* relationship between 'female' sex hormones (oestrogens and progestogens)[36] and premenstrual symptoms has *never* been demonstrated, only an association between the timing of symptoms and changes in their average circulating levels.[37] There are also no significant differences between the average levels of female sex hormones in the minority of those experiencing problematic cyclical symptoms and the majority who do not.[38] In fact, modern contraceptive medications containing both oestrogen and progestogen hormones are one of the first-line treatment options for *managing* premenstrual symptoms.[39]

While there is some evidence that individuals with underlying psychological distress are more likely to experience low or anxious mood when using hormonal contraceptive medications,[40] it is unclear if this is due to the synthetic hormones; other active substances in the pills; physiological changes brought about by use of the medications; or due to other factors in their mood state.[41] I argue, therefore, that until someone proves a *causal* relationship between any given hormone and low or anxious mood or cyclical symptoms in general, it would be best not to describe them as 'hormonal'. In addition, it would be more accurate to reframe the 'female' sex hormones as necessary for the coordination of important reproductive processes (in female *and* male bodies),[42] and as typically health promoting rather than inherently problematic or pathological chemicals.

The menstrual cycle as a series of inflammatory events

If not our hormones, what *can* account for our experiences of cyclical changes? From the early 1980s, physiologists (largely working in infertility research) have characterised the menstrual cycle as essentially *inflammatory* in nature. The three main events; ovulation – when an egg bursts out of an ovary;[43] SD – the regular thickening and decidualisation of the womb lining;[44] and menstruation – the loss of womb contents if no viable pregnancy is present,[45] were all found to involve cells, substances and processes indicative of an immune system response.[46] As a result, a growing body of research has developed regarding the potential role of healthy (and abnormal) cyclic inflammation in a range of fertility[47] and menstrual disorders, especially Polycystic Ovary Syndrome,[48] heavy menstrual bleeding,[49] endometriosis[50] and gynaecological cancers.[51]

So, it is very surprising that the PMS literature does not tend to mention inflammation.[52] Especially since common premenstrual changes directly reflect its cardinal signs (first identified by Celsus, way back in the 1st century AD): pain (*dolor*), heat (*calor*), redness/blood flow changes (*rubor*) and swelling/water retention (*tumor*).[53] Inflammation is also known to indirectly cause irritable and low mood states, fatigue, appetite changes, reduced sociability and reduced sleep quality.[54] What is more, inflammation appears to trigger or worsen a range of health issues, including those that can occur on a cyclic basis, such as asthma,[55] migraine,[56] epilepsy,[57] depression[58] and anxiety.[59]

Perhaps most importantly, a few population studies have shown that people experiencing problematic premenstrual symptoms have higher levels of inflammatory markers than those who do not.[60] For instance, Ellen Gold and colleagues sampled the blood of a diverse group of women participating in the US Study of Women's Health Across the Nation research project, 'a longitudinal, multicentre, multiracial/-ethnic study of midlife women'.[61] Those who reported problematic premenstrual mood symptoms, abdominal cramps, back pain, appetite cravings, weight gain, bloating and breast pain, were found to have elevated hs-CRP levels (a type of inflammatory protein).

Understanding that the second half of the menstrual cycle is inflammatory also fits extremely well with the available data regarding problematic premenstrual symptoms and their management. For instance, the diverse range of first-line treatments currently promoted for the treatment of PMS,[62] *all* have some sort of anti-inflammatory effect: exercise,[63] Cognitive Behavioural Therapy,[64] Vitamin B6,[65] drospirenone-containing hormonal contraceptive medications,[66] and selective serotonin reuptake inhibitors.[67] Similarly, anti-inflammatory medications, such as naproxen or ibuprofen (or dietary supplements such as Omega 3 fish oils[68]), taken 2–4 days before a period starts, can significantly reduce average menstrual blood loss (by about a third!), period pain and other premenstrual changes.[69]

Inflammation can also explain how external stressors influence premenstrual symptoms (and vice versa)[70] because inflammation is thought to mediate a two-way relationship between psychological and social experiences, and biological changes.[71] Finally, it also fits with the theory that SD and periods evolved to detect and destroy dangerous or unviable pregnancies, given its association with immune system processes. In short, there is plenty of available (yet largely ignored) evidence to support the idea that premenstrual changes are inflammatory, and *not* hormonal, in nature.

Menstrual blood loss and iron deficiency (anaemia)

Another likely factor in why some people experience problematic cyclical symptoms is iron deficiency. Iron levels are substantially affected by the blood loss associated with regular periods (approximately 20 litres or 44 pints over 40 years), plus childbirth (approximately 250ml per uncomplicated vaginal birth and one litre per uncomplicated caesarean section).[72] If iron deficient, heavier menstrual bleeding occurs, which in turn worsens the deficiency, creating a vicious cycle of negative physiological events.[73]

Shockingly, current clinical guidelines on the 'normal range' of circulating iron do not take female reproductive physiology into account. Instead, iron-deficiency anaemia is *mathematically* calculated as 'two standard deviations below' the *average* haemoglobin (Hb) level by 'age and sex' and reproductive status.[74] We already know that menstruation, pregnancy and childbirth are the most common causes of iron loss. Setting a lower 'normal range' simply because a population has lower average circulating levels does not mean that this population is healthy.[75] For example, right up until 2021, US clinical guidelines gave an even lower cut-off point for anaemia diagnoses in pregnant Black women, after they were found to have lower average iron levels. This was only stopped when it was discovered that these women had a 65 per cent higher chance of giving birth with anaemia (a known factor in maternal mortality).[76] Frustratingly, fixing the problem is not even hard or expensive! Dietary iron supplementation is a highly effective treatment for anaemia and is not subject to patent protection (making it very affordable).[77] This situation is a clear example of structural sexism and racism within medicine and wider society.[78]

In any case, given that a large proportion of the menstruating population is iron deficient, if not technically anaemic,[79] and this can cause a range of symptoms very similar to those associated with PMS,[80] iron status ought to be a key factor to investigate. To the best of my knowledge, however, only three clinical studies have *ever* investigated iron levels and premenstrual symptoms, and their findings all suggest a positive association between iron deficiency and common PMS symptoms.[81]

Again, it seems as though inflammation and iron deficiency (which really should be fairly obvious factors in menstrual health) have somehow been 'overlooked' in favour of hormonal explanations. Based on the findings of my PMS study (discussed in the second part of this book), I strongly suspect that the reduction of menstrual cycle physiology to its hormonal coordination within Western education has severely limited biomedical knowledge and practice over the past century. It appears 'hormonal fluctuations' have become equated with what 'the menstrual cycle' is, and all physiological events and experiences beyond them are, thus, obscured and made *mysterious*.[82] Unfortunately, because the word 'hormonal' also exists outside biomedical science as a euphemism for irrational behaviour (especially in women), the reduction of menstrual physiology to just its hormonal coordination also perpetuates sexist beliefs.

Think about how different things might have been if you had been fully informed about menstrual physiology from childhood: your first period or that of others, facing school exams, participating in sports, experiences of gender-based bullying or exclusion, seeking medical advice, making decisions about sex and sexual partners, making decisions about getting married or having children, making decisions about jobs, making decisions about how to inform and parent your own children, and the way you even feel about your body or that of your parent, partner, friend or child? These are not trivial things. Where ignorance exists, stigmatising myths thrive. Unless we address these gaps in our collective knowledge, efforts to improve gender equality in health and wider society are unlikely to succeed.

Box 1.1: The reduction and mystification of the menstrual cycle: why this matters

Science

Sadly, supposedly scientific biomedical discourses have (unintentionally) perpetuated societal gender (and at times, also racial) myths due to confirmation bias, rather than reflecting the available data. Think of the many fruitless investigations into the role of the female sex hormones in cyclical symptoms and other female-prevalent conditions. Not only were they a waste of scarce financial and human resources, but the consistently negative results which should have, but did not, put an end to the myth of the *hormonal* female, only seemed to reinforce yet another one; that of the *mysterious* female. This second myth is inherently anti-science, as well as sexist, in that it positions the female body as somehow beyond the reach of scientific knowledge and investigation. Given that women's health research is already disproportionately underfunded,[83] and especially so for Black and other racialised population groups,[84] implying that the female reproductive body is scientifically unknown/unknowable is unlikely to encourage fairer funding decisions in the future.

Clinical practice

The second part of this book describes the way in which this gap in knowledge has resulted in inadequate clinical research and practice regarding the diagnosis and treatment of PMS. However, nearly a century of perpetuating the 'hormonal female' myth within medicine and school education has wider clinical implications, too. Women in general (and Black and other racialised women in particular) are more likely to be met with medical disbelief, late diagnosis, misdiagnosis and the inadequate treatment of their symptoms (especially pain).[85] The societal stereotype of the 'hormonal/ hysterical' female (and racialised Other) must surely contribute to this situation. Many women wait over a decade to be diagnosed with debilitating conditions such as endometriosis[86] or Premenstrual Dysphoric Disorder,[87] and even then are not guaranteed prompt or effective treatment. Tellingly, our accounts of severe cyclic pain are often psychologised and positioned as 'normal' or 'all in our minds',[88] strongly suggestive that the myth of the hysterical/irrational female is still very much alive and well.

Society

Given that sexist societal depictions of the hysterical/hormonal female have been used to argue against women's right to vote, equal access to paid work, equal pay, leadership positions and agency over our own bodies,[89] this is a nasty stereotype to perpetuate, even unintentionally. If all we know of the menstrual cycle is its hormonal coordination, it is little wonder that the changes we experience are assumed to be hormonal in origin or that women in general are so easily positioned as hormonal in *essence*.

Similarly, by not teaching children or medical practitioners about the purpose of menstruation, research studies, clinical interactions, and political beliefs and policies are influenced by the erroneous assumption that the female body is only 'for' having children. Such pro-natalist bias has resulted in harmful restrictions on what is considered the proper moral behaviour for women,[90] as well as the clinical and physiological positioning of miscarriage as a 'failed pregnancy' rather than the 'successful termination of an unviable or potentially dangerous pregnancy'.[91] In fact, why did we switch from saying *spontaneous abortion* to the word *miscarriage* in the first place? The word essentially blames the woman/parent for something that is most likely due to a problem with an embryo or its placental attachment to the womb. Things beyond our control.

Personal

This brings me to the very personal implications of this gap in our education. Imagine the difference between being told that your difficulty in conceiving, or experiences of miscarriage, were most likely unviable pregnancies and beneficial for your own health and survival, rather than due to a faulty womb, or your behaviours during pregnancy? Imagine the difference between being told that your cyclic changes are inflammatory and relatively easily managed in most cases (unless there is an underlying health condition), rather than 'hormonal' and requiring more powerful, stigmatising or expensive medications (perhaps even surgery), plus the unhelpful and sexist connotation of being 'all in your mind' or somehow *caused by* your femininity?

2

How did we get here?

It might seem incredible that Western medicine can still be influenced by gender myths in 2025. But the myth of the hormonal/irrational female has a surprisingly long history, given that hormones were only first discovered around the turn of the last century. To provide some context to the origin of this myth and its association with the Premenstrual Syndrome (PMS) diagnosis, it is first necessary to briefly outline the history of a much older concept, *hysteria*.

It is worth noting that scholarly accounts of hysteria are typically split into two types: portrayals of a female prevalent biomedical condition, gradually revealing its true (biological/psychological) cause over time,[1] versus critical narratives of hysteria as an ever-changing diagnostic label more reflective of gender myths than a discrete pathological entity.[2] For this reason, both types of account are summarised separately in this chapter. However, my work aims to integrate biomedical and critical perspectives on hysteria and PMS by focusing on symptom type, which also allows an original argument to be made: that the diagnostic label of hysteria appears to have functioned in part to account for the *female prevalence* of certain symptoms and conditions.

Building on this argument, the second half of the chapter outlines the ways in which the diagnosis of PMS has come to be seen as 'the daughter of hysteria'.[3] Especially in respect to how PMS exists as both a biomedical condition *and* a widely accepted gender stereotype, and how its symptoms and sufferers are often met with disbelief and moral judgement. The chapter ends with a summary of why a critical analysis of the history of women's health is, therefore, necessary if we are ever to break out of the unintentional reproduction of gender and racial myths in clinical research and practice.

Female-prevalent symptoms throughout the history of medicine

Did you know that female-specific and prevalent symptoms have been recognised by physicians for at least the past 3,800 years? And that for the same length of time, they have been attributed to the reproductive body? We happen to know this because one of the oldest surviving written texts, the *Kahun Gynaecological Papyrus* (c. 1800 BCE), describes several such symptoms (uterine pain, heavy menstrual bleeding, headache and lower back pain) and ascribes them to 'discharges ... clenches ... wrappings

… or wandering of the womb'.[4] Similarly, Ancient Greek medical texts (c. 450–350 BCE) attribute 'all diseases of women' to the womb.[5] Either through the 'wandering' womb falling onto other organs,[6] or its 'suffocation' (denoting a lack of regular menstruation).[7] Crucially, most experiences listed are gynaecological in nature but other non-sex-specific symptoms, such as 'leg pain … headache … backache … breathlessness … seizures … and toothache', are also attributed to the womb, if affecting a woman.[8]

In this way, these texts exemplify a recurring theme in descriptions of female health throughout the history of Western medicine. The attribution of otherwise unexplained female-prevalent (including non-gynaecological) symptoms to whatever is currently positioned as *the* defining feature of embodied femininity.[9] For most of recorded history, this was the womb and because the Ancient Greek word for womb was *Hyster*, such symptoms were often described as 'hysteria'. Contrary to popular belief, however, eminent medical historian, Helen King, has shown that ancient hysterical symptoms were *exclusively* physical in nature, and they remained so until relatively recently.[10] Indeed, it was not until the 16th century that Western accounts of hysteria first began to refer to emotional symptoms.[11]

In the 17th century, a physician called Thomas Sydenham purposefully redefined hysteria as a specific type of disease rather than a general explanation for women's symptoms. Sydenham defined hysteria as a female-prevalent (but not sex-specific) *nervous condition*, citing the 'weaker constitution' of the female body as a cause of 'emotional instability'.[12] He also positioned emotional distress as a potential *cause* of hysteria (which could present as numerous physical symptoms, including gastrointestinal pain, severe headache or migraine, and recurrent abdominal and muscular pain).[13] Importantly, Sydenham directly compared the diverse physical and emotional symptoms of hysteria to those observed in *hypochondriasis*, defined at the time as a male prevalent form of *melancholia* (low mood) associated with a range of physical complaints, and thought to be caused by an 'obstruction of the spleen'.[14]

> As to females, if we except those who lead a hard and hardy life, there is rarely one who is wholly free from it [hysteria]. … Then, again, such male subjects as lead a sedentary or studious life, and grow pale over their books and papers, are similarly afflicted; since however much antiquity may have laid the blame of hysteria upon the uterus, hypochondriasis … is as like it, as one egg is to another.[15]

In short, the same types of symptoms were given a different diagnostic label and biological source if affecting men or women (even though women were known to have spleens, too)! In an apparent attempt to explain the female prevalence of such symptoms, Sydenham also proposed (without evidence) that female hysteria was much more common than its male counterpart due to an inherent *weakness* of constitution in all (except the hardiest of) women. Between the 17th and 19th centuries, however, the meaning of *hypochondriasis* shifted to reflect the concepts with which it is associated today; imagined, exaggerated or consciously fabricated illness and/or an obsessive preoccupation with one's health. Since the diagnosis of hysteria was already associated with hypochondria, this meant that female-prevalent symptoms also became *questionable* in terms of their perceived reality or biomedical legitimacy: 'These patients are veritable actresses; they do not know of a greater pleasure than to deceive. ... The hysterics who exaggerate their convulsive movement ... make an equal travesty and exaggeration of the movements of their soul, their ideas and their acts. ... In one word, the life of the hysteric is nothing but one perpetual falsehood.'[16]

By the end of the 19th century, the highly influential work of Sigmund Freud had firmly recategorised hysteria as a type of *psychological neurosis* caused by (sexual) trauma.[17] This new definition positioned otherwise unexplained physical symptoms as primarily *caused by* emotional distress.[18] Consequently, hysterical symptoms continued to be directly associated with 'imagined illness', in both biomedical and popular discourses. While Freud explicitly separated the diagnosis of hysteria from the womb, his theories did imply categorical sex differences between men and women's psychologies and brain development, in part to explain the relative female prevalence of symptoms. In this way, Freud's definition of hysteria continued the ancient tradition of citing the essence of femininity as the ultimate cause of otherwise unexplained female-prevalent symptoms, just substituting the womb for the 'female psyche'.

While most historical accounts of hysteria agree that it essentially *disappeared* as a clinical diagnosis and embodied experience in the early 20th century, biomedical explanations as for why this happened are typically vague and unsubstantiated. For instance, Micale simply states: 'After twenty centuries of medical history, this extraordinary disease is for all intents and purposes disappearing from sight today. Nobody knows why.'[19] Writing in the 1960s, Veith attributed its sudden disappearance to the success of Freudian psychoanalytic therapy:

> Freud's studies on hysteria, instead of endowing this illness with greater significance, actually divested it of much of the mystical importance it held for more than two millennia. ... The newly gained insight into therapy finds its application in the severe neuroses in general within which the potential hysterics of today are presumably included.[20]

What is hinted at in Veith's final sentence is perhaps a more compelling biomedical explanation; that the boom in psychological therapy created new labels for specific types of neuroses, thus, the entity previously known as 'hysteria' still existed, just under different names.

Medical historians seem to have completely overlooked another possible factor in the demise of hysteria, however. Several *physical* symptoms previously regarded as common expressions of the diagnosis may also have been given alternative diagnostic labels after hysteria was reclassified as a psychological disorder in the late 19th century.[21] For instance, digestive symptoms may have been alternatively diagnosed as *spastic colon* (later renamed *irritable bowel syndrome*); visual disturbances and severe headaches as *migraine*; seizures as *epilepsy*; muscular and joint pain as *fibrositis* (later renamed *fibromyalgia*); chronic fatigue as ME (*Myalgic Encephalomyelitis*); and lethargy, loss of appetite, difficulty swallowing, pallor, breathlessness and fainting as iron-deficiency *anaemia*.

Crucially, these conditions are female prevalent (except for epilepsy), medically unexplained (except for anaemia) and, thus, subject to clinical and societal disbelief,[22] making them also somewhat 'hysterical/hypochondriacal' in all but name. In other words, while we may no longer have a biomedical classification called hysteria, Western medicine has simply split female-prevalent physical and emotional symptoms into different groupings, while maintaining underlying assumptions about them being wholly or partially psychologically induced, and in some way *caused by* embodied femininity.

Key political and philosophical influences on female hysteria

Let us turn to more critical accounts of hysteria. The tendency to assign female-prevalent symptoms without an obvious cause to whichever entity is currently positioned as the essence of femininity has likely been contested for millennia. Not least, because most women have female bodies but do not experience debilitating symptoms, and so the empirical inconsistency of such theories is likely to have been noticed. In addition, the idea of a literally 'wandering' pathological womb was contested from the start, and by highly influential physicians such as Soranus of Ephesus (c. 80–138 AD) and Galen (c. 129–216 AD).[23] Yet, it was not until the resurgence of human anatomy in the 17th century that the notion of the wandering womb was finally quashed. The truth lay exposed for all to see upon the dissection table; 'the womb ... is so strictly tied by neighbouring parts round about, that it cannot of itself be moved, or ascend from its place'.[24] In fact, over 350 years ago, the anatomist and physician Thomas Willis (a contemporary and rival of Thomas Sydenham) eloquently and succinctly expressed the same argument that I make here.

The hysterical passion is of so ill fame among the diseases belonging to women, that like one half damn'd, it bears the faults of many distempers: For when at any time a sickness happens in a woman's body, of an unusual manner ... so that its causes lie hid, and a curatory indication is altogether uncertain, presently we accuse the evil influence of the womb (which for the most part is innocent) and in every unusual symptom, we declare it to be something hysterical and so to this scope, which oftentimes is only the subterfuge of ignorance, the medical intentions and use of remedies are directed.[25]

More recently, hysteria has been positioned as an example of a socially constructed disease, which served to legitimise and maintain patriarchal, White supremacist and capitalist societal interests.[26] Since the 1990s postmodern turn in academia, critical historical,[27] philosophical,[28] literary[29] and sociological[30] scholars have persuasively argued that the ever-changing diagnosis of hysteria primarily reflected societal concerns about the political status of women (and certain men deemed inferior based on their perceived effeminacy, occupation, race, sexuality, class or mental/physical debility). This perspective helps to explain why the assumed causes of hysteria were constantly shifting over time, yet always implied a specifically feminine biological pathology. The diagnosis of hysteria, thus, formalised pre-existing societal stereotypes that positioned femininity (and other characteristics deemed 'inferior', such as a racialised or colonised ethnicity) as a form of mental and physical debility or illness.

For instance, Sydenham added emotional distress to the previously gynaecological diagnosis of hysteria at a time of immense social change, which had a profound impact on gender relations and the political position of women.[31] Related to these changes was the development of a new Western European philosophical ideal, 'The Man of Reason', identified by Genevieve Lloyd.[32] Descartes' famous dualist method of reasoning transformed some of Classical philosophy's binary pairings, that positioned the relation between men/women as being *symbolic* of reason/emotion, master/slave and culture/nature, into much more literal beliefs.[33] In this way, the intellectual ideal of 'The Man of Reason' simultaneously created an implied opposite construct, 'The Emotional/Irrational Woman' (and/or colonised populations, or slaves).[34]

Descartes' *Discours de la méthode*, was published just 30 years before Sydenham first associated hysteria with excessive emotion.[35] Given the alleged binary opposition between reason and emotion, this philosophical and societal context is also the likely origin of another gender/race myth; that women/racialised Others are 'biologically' prone to irrational behaviour, and, consequently, that female-prevalent or otherwise unexplained symptoms in women and racialised Others may simply be 'all in the mind'. A myth likely reinforced by hysteria's direct association with hypochondriasis (which was soon to become synonymous with imagined or invented illness).

Similarly, as Silvia Federici eloquently argued, changing gender relations in the Early Modern period were inextricably linked to the advent of capitalism, since it required the 'separation of production from reproduction'.[36] It is reasonable to suggest that the shift in biomedical descriptions of hysteria at this time may have also reflected a capitalist need to *naturalise* unequal political power. Especially given that the diagnosis of hysteria reinforced the idea that women (and colonised men/slaves) were physically, emotionally or mentally unfit for waged work (as opposed to unpaid or very low paid labour, which was deemed their *natural* role). Indeed, the label of hysteria was later frequently applied to women participating in the suffrage movement,[37] and in the United States, an associated disorder – *drapetomania* – was a legitimate biomedical diagnosis reserved for Black slaves (but not White servants) who ran away from their masters.[38] Diagnoses such as hysteria have, therefore, been used to challenge deviation from imposed social roles and to argue that such roles were 'natural', and for the good of one's health rather than in the interest of patriarchal, White supremacist, colonial, slave labour-dependent, capitalist societies.[39]

In fact, as beautifully explained by Nancy Stepan, by the mid-19th century, various Western European 'sciences' strongly associated with colonial expansion (such as anthropology, phrenology and biology) were *explicitly* comparing women's bodies and, especially their minds and brains, with those of racialised colonial subjects, criminals and the lower classes.[40] While these sexist, racist and classist beliefs have now been disproven and rejected by most research scientists, the pseudoscientific political use of biological data to try and *justify* systematic social discrimination and oppression continues to this day.[41]

> By the 1850s, the measurement of women's skulls was becoming an established part of craniometry and the science of gender joined analogically to race. Vogt's Lectures on Man included a long discussion of the various measures available of the skulls of men and women of different races. His data showed that women's smaller brains were analogous to the brains of lower races, the small size explaining both groups' intellectual inferiority. (Vogt also concluded that within Europe the intelligentsia and upper classes had the largest heads, and peasants the smallest).[42]

It is worth noting that critical scholars do not insist that the individual men of medicine who, with hindsight, seem to have acted complicitly with discriminatory practices and rhetoric, were conscious of doing so, or even necessarily held such beliefs (although Freud was demonstrably anti-suffragist[43]). For instance, Sydenham could not have known that hypochondriasis would eventually change its meaning, thus associating hysteria (and femininity itself) with imagined, exaggerated or fabricated symptoms. The point is that medicine cannot help but *reflect* societal beliefs, even when it aims for scientific objectivity, because it is carried out by individuals who are typically unaware of their own cultural assumptions and biases.[44]

Critical arguments do not deny it is possible that more women experience emotional distress than men. They simply claim that emotional distress is more likely a result of distressing events and experiences, than the healthy functioning of the female body.[45] Certainly, another factor in the demise of hysteria as a biomedical diagnosis was the visibility of male-prevalent illnesses connected to the First World War. Thousands of returning soldiers exhibited the same signs of *hysteria* previously associated with the womb and female psyche. Given that these men did not possess such things, their expressions of extreme emotional distress and unexplained physical symptoms could no longer be attributed to embodied femininity. They were ultimately given another diagnostic label, *shell shock*, which became a pejorative term as the condition was swiftly equated with cowardice and physical/moral/ psychological weakness.[46] Yet again, medically unexplained symptoms were positioned as imagined or invented, a sign of immorality, and distinctly un-masculine (that is, feminine/hysterical), even in men who had clearly experienced traumatic events.

From hysterical to hormonal: the emergence of biomedical PMS

Just as female hysteria began to disappear, the sex hormones were discovered. Oestrogen was first identified in 1929 and the very same year, a US gynaecologist called Robert Frank wrote a handbook on female sex hormones.[47] The cover of his book bore a Latin inscription, '*propter secretions internas totas, mulier est quod est*', meaning 'because of her internal secretions, the woman is what she is'.[48] Crucially, Frank also wrote the first formal description of Premenstrual Tension (PMT) a couple of years later, in 1931.[49] His paper documented cases of cyclical asthma attacks, epileptic fits, water retention, and cardiac irregularity, but its focus was on the experiences of a small subset of patients, characterised by various signs of 'nervous tension' (Table 2.1).[50] Frank attributed all cyclic symptoms to an *excess* of the female hormone (oestrogen) (later disproven).[51]

Note how Robert Frank describes his patients (Table 2.1). He reports the number of children and abortions (miscarriages) each patient has had. Un/successful motherhood was clearly something Frank was interested in recording, probably because he felt it was relevant to the PMT diagnosis. Several of the *complaints* also appear to be value judgements rather than symptoms; 'unbearable', 'shrew', 'almost crazy', 'sexual tension' and 'impossible to live with'. Finally, we can see how he attributed PMT to an excess of oestrogen (the new essence of femininity), since the recommended treatment options are either applying radiation to, or surgically removing,

Table 2.1: Cases of Premenstrual Tension

	Age	Regular menses	Parity		Complaints	Relief with onset of menses	Treatment
			Chil-dren	Abor-tions			
R.P.	35	+	2	1	Severest tension; double oophorectomy advised elsewhere	Immediate	X-ray 'toning'
B.H.	32	+	2	1	Severest tension; suicidal desire	Immediate	X-ray 'toning'
F.B.	41	+	3	0	Severest tension; unbearable, shrew	Gradual	
L.H.	47	+	2	0	Severest tension; husband to be pitied	Immediate	Elimination
M.M.	28	+	0	0	Severest tension; suicidal desire	After 1 day	
A.B.	38	+	4	3	Severest tension; 'almost crazy'	Immediate	X-rays advised
H.C.	35	+	1	1	Severest tension; psychoneurotic	Immediate	
B.M.	38	+	Unmarried		Severe tension; incapacitated mentally	Immediate	Elimination
K.R.	43	+	2	1	Severe tension; sexual tension, also	Toward end of period	
M.L.	33	+	1	0	Severe tension; cardiac irregularity	Gradual	Elimination
A.W.	41	+	2	1	Severe tension; 'impossible to live with'	Immediate	
B.N.	32	+	1	0	Moderate tension; despondent	Immediate	
E.M.	35	+	3	0	Moderate tension	Immediate	
C.R.	33	+	2	0	Moderate tension	Immediate	
S.S.	24	+	0	0	Moderate tension	Immediate	

Source: Adapted from Frank (1931)

the ovaries. These discursive patterns are extremely reminiscent of 19th-century accounts of female hysteria.[52]

Interestingly, hormones were also swiftly integrated into biological essentialist justifications for colonisation and racism. Nancy Stepan neatly summarises how gender and racial myths were co-created and explained in reference to each other, and an assumed shared 'hormonal' biological inferiority:

> A last confirmatory example of the … [political analogy between] gender and race … is taken from the history of hormone biology. Early in the twentieth century … Sir Arthur Keith interpreted racial differences in the human species as a function of pathological disturbances of the newly discovered 'internal secretions' or hormones. … At about the same time … Havelock Ellis used internal secretions to explain the … vital differences in the physical and psychosexual makeup of men and women. In short, lower races represented the 'female' type of the human species, and females the 'lower race' of gender.[53]

From the 1950s, Katharina Dalton, a UK-based private general practitioner (GP), was instrumental in changing the name and concept of PMT (Premenstrual Tension) to PMS (Premenstrual Syndrome), arguing that premenstrual symptoms were more physical in nature than just nervous tension.[54] Alas, while this one aspect of her work challenged the 'psychologisation' of female-prevalent symptoms, Dalton also reinforced several other gender myths in her work. For instance, she cited a highly exaggerated total of 150 premenstrual symptoms,[55] even though the vast majority listed were indicative of underlying health conditions triggered or worsened by the menstrual cycle.[56] Dalton also claimed that 'nearly half of all women' suffered from debilitating PMS; that it had a highly detrimental effect on women's ability to work as well as reducing the productivity of their husbands; and that it caused violent and other criminal behaviours.[57] These incredible claims, however, were exclusively based on 'low quality anecdotal accounts'.[58] Dalton also attributed cyclic symptoms to a female sex hormone, only this time it was a *deficiency* in progesterone (later disproven).[59]

Gao and colleagues have helpfully synthesised all PMS-related publications between 1950 and 2018 (Figure 2.1).[60] Spot the sharp increase in the number of PMS papers from 1981. This was the year that Katharina Dalton acted as an expert witness in two murder cases. Her testimony argued that PMS had rendered the defendants 'not responsible' for their actions, which resulted in significantly reduced sentencing and attracted a high level of media and scholarly attention.[61] You may be relieved to hear that a subsequent review of the available data on menstruation and crime found no evidence of a relationship between criminal action of any sort with any phase of the menstrual cycle![62]

Figure 2.1: Publications on premenstrual disorders per year, 1950–2018

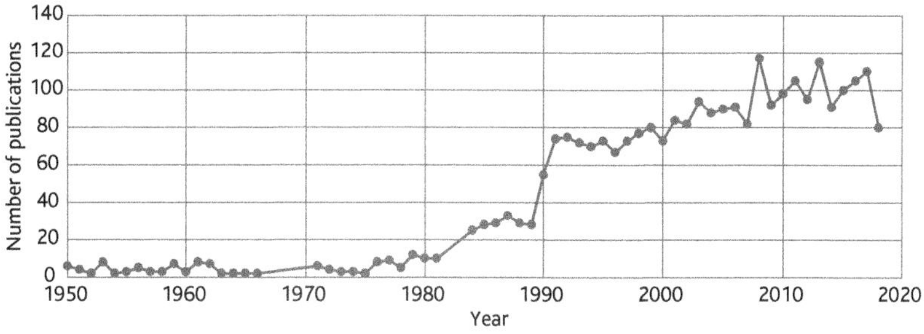

Source: Adapted from Gao et al (2021)

Another spike in PMS research publications occurred around 1990 (Figure 2.1), following the inclusion of a new premenstrual condition, Late Luteal Phase Dysphoric Disorder (LLPDD), in the 1987 American Psychiatric Association's list of diagnoses.[63] LLPDD was later renamed PMDD (Premenstrual Dysphoric Disorder). Please note the inclusion of several common and non-pathological cyclic changes (fatigue, changes in appetite, breast swelling, bloating, muscle pain and weight gain) in the diagnostic criteria of this *psychiatric* condition (Table 2.2). As a result of these two pivotal events, biomedical descriptions of PMS reverted to being predominantly mood-based in the early 1980s.[64]

So where are we now when it comes to biomedical definitions of PMS? Let us take a look at the latest Royal College of Obstetricians and Gynaecologists (RCOG) clinical guidelines.

> PMS encompasses a *vast array of psychological symptoms* such as depression, anxiety, irritability, loss of confidence and mood swings. There are also physical symptoms, typically bloatedness [*sic*] and mastalgia [breast pain]. *It is the timing, rather than the types of symptoms*, and the degree of impact on daily activity that supports a diagnosis of PMS. *The character of symptoms in an individual patient does not influence the diagnosis.*[65]

Contrary to the available population data,[66] the current RCOG definition positions PMS as more of a psychological than pain-based experience. The definition is also highly unusual in that it simultaneously suggests that *any* premenstrual symptom counts, so long as it is significantly impairing. No other diagnosis is similarly based on the *timing* of any symptoms rather than any causal explanation or otherwise deterministic, or even most common, list of associated symptoms. In fact, when it comes to a causal explanation for PMS, the RCOG guidelines get even more interesting: 'Although the aetiology (cause) remains uncertain, it revolves around the ovarian hormone

Table 2.2: A–D of the diagnostic criteria for PMDD in DSM V

A	In the majority of menstrual cycles, at least five symptoms must be present in the final week before the onset of menses, start to improve within a few days after the onset of menses, and become minimal or absent in the week post menses.
B	One (or more) of the following symptoms must be present: 1. Marked affective lability (e.g., mood swings: feeling suddenly sad or tearful, or increased sensitivity to rejection). 2. Marked irritability or anger or increased interpersonal conflicts. 3. Marked depressed mood, feelings of hopelessness, or self-deprecating thoughts. 4. Marked anxiety, tension, and/or feelings of being keyed up or on edge.
C	One (or more) of the following symptoms must additionally be present, to reach a total of five symptoms when combined with symptoms from Criterion B above: 5. Decreased interest in usual activities (e.g., work, school, friends, hobbies). 6. Subjective difficulty in concentration. 7. Lethargy, easy fatigability, or marked lack of energy. 8. Marked change in appetite; overeating; or specific food cravings. 9. Hypersomnia or insomnia. 10. A sense of being overwhelmed or out of control. 11. Physical symptoms such as breast tenderness or swelling, joint or muscle pain, a sensation of 'bloating,' or weight gain.
Note:	The symptoms in Criteria A–C must have been met for most menstrual cycles that occurred in the preceding year.
D	The symptoms are associated with clinically significant distress or interference with work, school, usual social activities, or relationships with others (e.g., avoidance of social activities; decreased productivity and efficiency at work, school, or home).

Source: APA (2013)

cycle. … [Although] the serum concentrations of oestrogen or progesterone are the same in those with or without PMS.'[67] Immediately after stating that the cause remains uncertain (that is, due to a lack of evidence and the fact there is no difference in hormone levels between those with or without symptoms), the 'ovarian hormone cycle' is still confidently implicated as the cause of PMS.[68] As discussed throughout this book, it seems as though pervasive gender myths, and a lack of adequate medical education in healthy menstrual physiology, play a major part in perpetuating this type of circular logic. Why else would biomedical descriptions of PMS continue to position the female sex hormones as pathological, despite decades of contradictory research findings?

The emergence of critical perspectives on PMS

Only a few months after Robert Frank first formally described PMT, Karen Horney, a renowned German psychoanalyst, published an alternative analysis.[69] Horney proposed that the normal and healthy physiological changes involved in the menstrual cycle were subconsciously noticed, and in some individuals, symbolically associated with 'a preparation for pregnancy'.[70] This could then prompt emotional distress in individuals who felt conflicted in some way about motherhood. Crucially, Horney explicitly positioned this psychological theory as directly opposing Frank's hormonal theory: 'I want once more to mark the boundaries of this concept as against that of the gynaecologists. ... We are not dealing with a basic weakness, a condition leading to the ... lesser efficiency of women.'[71]

Frank and Horney were writing just 20 years after some women had first been granted the right to vote in US/German parliamentary elections. They were, therefore, both likely to have been aware of one of the main arguments used against women's suffrage; that women were mentally unfit to make an informed and rational voting decision due to their female (reproductive) body (that is, the myth of the inherently irrational hysterical female).[72] This context helps to explain Horney's immediate reaction to Frank's paper, and her concern that a solely biological explanation for PMT risked swift societal extrapolation to 'all women'.

Much like the biomedical literature, however, critical perspectives on PMS only really took off in the early 1980s. The 'PMS defence' successfully used to mitigate murder charges against two women in 1981 prompted extensive media coverage. As several critical scholars pointed out, this coverage typically implied that 'all women' were potentially dangerous and 'out of control' before and during menstruation.[73] In fact, a PMS stereotype depiction of irrationally irritable and/or pathologically emotional 'hormonal' women became widely recognised and frequently cited in the popular media, jokes and even some biomedical resources.[74] This new PMS stereotype image was (and remains) strikingly similar to earlier depictions of the hysterical female (and suffragette) (Figure 2.2).

Biomedical, legal and critical health scholars criticised Dalton's 'PMS defence' as being unscientific, a dangerous unsubstantiated legal precedent, and biologically essentialist sexism.[75] By the time any link between criminal behaviour and the menstrual cycle had been thoroughly disproven, however, the US National Institute of Mental Health had already held an international conference to try and standardise the diagnostic criteria for (a predominantly mood-based) PMS,[76] and an American Psychiatric Association committee had been convened to develop diagnostic criteria for its inclusion in the Diagnostic and Statistical Manual of Mental Disorders (that is, as a specific premenstrual 'mental disorder').[77] It was at this point, during the mid-1980s, that PMS became *highly* contested by, and a substantial research interest for, critical health scholars.

PMS as a highly contested and gendered diagnosis

Medical sociologist, Anne Figert, identified three overlapping *domains* of this conflict ('science', 'health' and 'woman') in which various interest

Figure 2.2: Popular media images of the hysterical/hormonal female

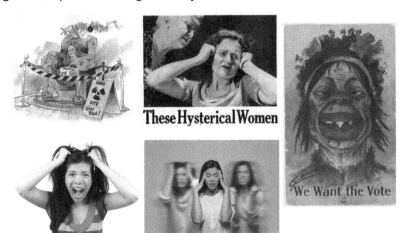

Source: (a) Ray Russotto, (b) Lidia Pinkham Tincture ad, public domain as seen https://vintage-ads.livejournal.com/1702922.html, (c) Anonymous, *We Want the Vote* (1908). Museum of London, image no. 010260. LSE Library; Museum of London Picture Library, (d) Adobe Stock/elnariz, (e) Adobe Stock/Maridav

groups have competed, to present and defend different accounts of PMS and PMDD.[78] Broadly speaking, in the 'science' domain, biomedical researchers have consistently tried yet failed to define diagnostic boundaries, identify a hormonal causal mechanism or develop any specific or universally effective (pharmaceutical) treatments for premenstrual disorders. Many other biomedical and critical health scholars have, therefore, questioned the scientific validity and legitimacy of the PMS and PMDD diagnoses.[79]

In the 'health' domain, gynaecologists, psychiatrists and (critical) experts have competed with one another for authoritative credibility and ownership of premenstrual symptoms (and, it has been argued, their considerable financial potential, particularly within the US private healthcare system). In the 'woman' domain, professional (biomedical and critical health scholars) and lay women (especially self-identified PMS sufferers) have made different *gendered* ownership claims about PMS. For instance, some psychiatrists positioned the LLPDD diagnostic category as countering gender myths, whereas for other psychiatrists, critical scholars and PMS sufferers, they were thought to reproduce them.[80]

This high level of contestation exists because without any proven biological (hormonal) cause, the biomedical labels of PMS and PMDD *must* represent something more than simply a physiological disease or abnormality. Critical scholars have, thus, been arguing since the 1980s that while premenstrual experiences are 'real', the biomedical labels of PMS and PMDD are culturally specific discourses.[81] For instance, the bulk of the biomedical literature on PMS/PMDD has come from the United States, then Western European

Table 2.3: The top ten countries publishing PMS/PMDD studies, 1945–2018

Rank	Country/Region	Count
1	United States	1,242
2	England	274
3	Sweden	194
4	Canada	174
5	Australia	140
6	Italy	125
7	Germany	100
8	Netherlands	77
9	Japan	74
10	People's Republic of China	62

Source: Adapted from Gao et al (2021)

nations and former British colonies, and only much more recently from China (Table 2.3).

The concept of PMS also *originated* in the United States and became a research interest in countries sharing the same Western biomedical model of disease, which typically ignores the social context of a patient in favour of purely biological explanations.[82] In many instances this is not a problem, but when no physical abnormality, dysfunction or disease can be identified, biomedical accounts may fail to consider other (environmental, psychological or social) factors in ill-health,[83] perhaps especially in the case of psychiatric diagnoses.[84] For PMS, as a sex-specific diagnosis, this includes a multitude of non-biological *gendered* (psychosocial) factors associated with being a woman within any given patriarchal society.[85]

Chrisler's cross-cultural PMS study also found that premenstrual symptoms vary by country and appear to reflect 'culture-bound' beliefs about femininity.[86] People in the UK are significantly more likely to report mood-related premenstrual symptoms than those living in several nearby countries, including France, Germany, Hungary, Italy and Spain.[87] Chinese women are unlikely to mention negative mood changes (unless prompted to do so by a symptom list[88]) but frequently describe 'feeling the cold',[89] something that is not typically described by women in the United States or Western Europe.[90] Indeed, prior to the 1980s, specifically 'pre' menstrual symptoms were rarely described by US patients,[91] and a study of immigrant and US-born Asian, Black and Latina women found that the longer the time exposed to US culture, the more likely an individual was to report premenstrual emotional distress.[92] It has been argued, therefore, that while female reproductive physiology is universal, 'what counts as PMS' is subject to cultural beliefs, discourses and practices.[93]

Similarly, several critical scholars have argued that 'what counts as PMS' may also serve a *moral* purpose.[94] Biomedical descriptions of PMS (like hysteria before it) appear in part to exert judgement and, thus, control over women's behaviour. For example, the inclusion of certain premenstrual symptoms in PMS diagnostic tools that are actually moral judgements on non-pathological and stereotypically 'feminine' human behaviours. Halbreich's consolidation of 200 behavioural descriptions (later reduced to 150), included dozens of such pseudo-symptoms, including 'act spiteful', 'tend to nag' or 'tend to blame others for problems'.[95] In other words, the US/Western European biomedical focus on premenstrual negative mood changes may reproduce predominantly US/Western European gender myths regarding the 'hysterical/ irrational female'.[96]

Accordingly, just as the label and concept of hysteria was used to justify and maintain patriarchal interests, critical scholars have argued that premenstrual diagnoses function in much the same way. For instance, Emily Martin and others, such as Sophie Laws[97] and Jane Ussher,[98] have suggested that the boom in public, clinical and academic interest in PMS since the early 1980s was partly in response to women's 'greater incursions into the paid work force' as a result of gains made in access to contraception, education and anti-discriminatory legislation brought about by second-wave feminism.[99] Certainly, the PMS stereotype reproduced in the popular media is often applied to the context of work, especially female leadership, or power within or beyond the home.[100] Tellingly, the PMS stereotype transcends reproductive status and is just as easily applied to menopausal women (Figure 2.3), or even the personification of femininity, herself, 'Mother Nature' (Figure 2.4).

In short, the PMS stereotype is very much the current incarnation of the hysterical female myth. Unfortunately, this means that physiological cyclical changes (mainly pain-related) are conceptually and linguistically (through the PMS label) linked to a 19th-century gender myth that positions them as predominantly 'psychological' in origin and essence.[101] What was once dismissed as 'hysterical' is now often dismissed as 'hormonal'. Both terms explain away the female prevalence of pain-related symptoms and emotional distress as being caused by femininity (either our bodies or our psyches), rather than other non-sex-specific factors, such as inflammation or distressing life experiences. Indeed, the assumption that women are 'hormonal' in essence (and men somehow are not!) has, without a doubt, contributed to the reduction of menstrual physiology to only its hormonal coordination in medical and school education.

While critical accounts of female hysteria and PMS do a great job at revealing social and political factors influencing both diagnoses, they also tend to overlook the female prevalence of certain symptoms.[103] Many women really do experience cyclic symptoms, mainly pain-related, but also changes in mood.[104] Several health conditions are also triggered or worsened

Figure 2.3: PMS as gender myth: Hilary Clinton depicted as pathologically emotional due to PMS during her party leadership campaign in 2007 (when she was 60 years old!)

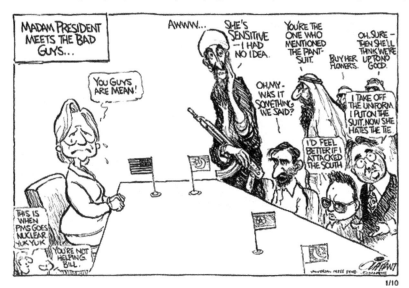

Figure 2.4: PMS as gender myth: 'Mother Nature' depicted as hysterical and subject to PMS (also despite being post-reproductive age in appearance), published in 2011

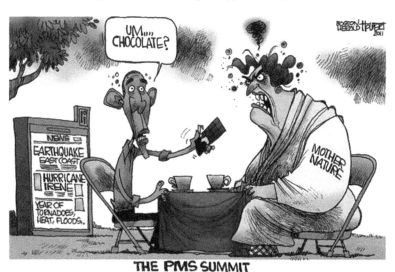

Source: Holbert, J. (2011, September 20) The PMS Summit [Cartoon] The Boston Herald. Reproduced with permission

during the second half of the menstrual cycle.[105] So how do we describe and investigate these experiences without unintentionally reproducing gender myths? In short, by applying the scientific method to ensure that everything we describe is actually supported by the available evidence.

The second part of this book outlines my doctoral research study, which compared expert and lay descriptions of PMS with the available population data on premenstrual symptoms. Spoiler alert! The participant descriptions are far more reflective of gender myths than the available data, but by analysing them I am able to make some recommendations for how we might avoid this pitfall in the future.

Box 2.1: From hysterical to hormonal: why this matters

Science

Blaming female-prevalent symptoms on whatever is currently considered the embodiment of femininity is not just bad science, it is a persistent and sexist biomedical assumption that needs to be exposed and challenged. It is time we stopped funding and carrying out research on 'hormonal' causes of female-prevalent symptoms, without sufficient proof of concept. Instead, we should fund and investigate more evidence-based psychosocial and biological explanations for the female prevalence of certain symptoms.

We must avoid the biomedical gendering of certain symptoms as 'feminine', simply because more women than men experience them, as this is a logical fallacy. Likewise, the female prevalence of many chronic health conditions is worth scientific investigation – it should not be considered 'normal' to be ill or to experience certain debilitating symptoms simply because you are a woman or have a female reproductive system. Biomedical diagnostic criteria should be based on indicators of health or illness, not mathematical calculations based on (socially stratified) sub-population averages.

The fact that most people experiencing severe emotional distress have experienced distressing things urgently needs to be integrated into scientific research into biological factors in poor mental and physical health, and not simply dismissed as insignificant, or paradoxically, 'unscientific' information. Not only can this approach help explain prevalence rate differences by sex, gender, ethnicity, disability, socioeconomic status or location, but it will likely bring valuable insights to our work.

Clinical practice

The myth of the hysterical/hormonal female or Other clearly influences the way in which women (and racialised and other socially marginalised population groups) are treated in clinical interactions, which can ultimately have a negative impact on our health outcomes. I have lost count of the number of people I have met who were initially (and sometimes repeatedly) told their debilitating pain was 'all in their head' or 'normal' or 'just part of being a woman'. Medical students need to be taught that we all hold these types of unconscious biases, and how to identify and challenge them in clinical practice.

Society

As critical scholars have been pointing out for a century, blaming female-prevalent symptoms on the essence of femininity (without adequate evidence) upholds, if not endorses, sexist beliefs in wider society. First 'all women' were hysterical, now we are hormonal (regardless of our actual health or reproductive status). We know that our bodies are not to blame for political inequalities, because most women are healthy and the same kinds of discourses are used against racialised, disabled, emotionally distressed, chronically ill, working-class and poor men, too. It is time to expose and eliminate the myth of the hysterical/hormonal/irrational female and Other, once and for all.

Personal

You might have sometimes described yourself as hormonal.[102] Please do not do this from now on! Your emotions and other cyclic changes are not caused by your sex hormones. They occur in response to annoying or upsetting situations and are merely worsened by various embodied states, such as pain, hunger, dehydration, tiredness, anaemia and systemic inflammation (including that associated with the menstrual cycle). Work out what is upsetting you and try to improve the situation, rather than endorsing the idea that the female sex hormones dictate our moods. The difference between attributing cyclic changes to iron deficiency and/or inflammation versus sex hormones is that the hormonal explanation is gendered and not based on the available evidence (and thus, sexist). There is less chance of perpetuating nasty 'all women' gender myths by using more accurate descriptions of what we experience.

PART II

Where are we now? PMS (Premenstrual Syndrome)

After reading the first part of this book, you should have more of an understanding of menstrual physiology beyond hormones, and why we got stuck on hormones in the first place. Now I hope to illustrate the way in which hormonal descriptions of the female reproductive body limit and stigmatise our understanding and experiences of female-prevalent symptoms. For this, we will use the example of Premenstrual Syndrome (PMS), the biomedical label applied to a range of experiences occurring during the second half (luteal/secretory phase) of the menstrual cycle.

I first started researching cyclical symptoms and associated gender myths over a decade ago. Having read much of the critical and biomedical literature on PMS while creating the Menstrual Matters website, I knew that it was possible to integrate supposedly oppositional critical and biomedical perspectives on menstrual health … because this is what I automatically did in my head! The problem was how to do so in a way that might persuade others working in this space (biomedical experts, critical experts, clinicians and patient-activists) that their different perspectives could complement rather than antagonise each other.

In my doctoral research, I also wanted to hear directly from people who experience cyclic symptoms. To strip away all the baggage attached to the research literature and get closer to what people actually feel, say and think about their menstrual health. This created various methodological and theoretical challenges, however. How could I meaningfully combine data and literatures from physiology, biology, epidemiology, critical theory, sociology, psychology and gender studies with the words and perspectives of patients? To be honest, identifying a practical and robust research methodology took a while and involved a lot of dead ends. The good news is that you do not have to read all about those and can instead go straight to the part where I worked out how to do it, did it, and what I found out!

This first chapter provides an overview of what I did and why. The following four chapters discuss each of the major themes identified in the interview data. The concluding chapter brings these findings together, before ending with an urgent call to action regarding menstrual health literacy.

Remember! If you find any part of this book to be too detailed or academic for your taste, you can always skip to the chapter summary and 'Why this matters' box at the end of each chapter. This will tell you all you really need to know.

3

What counts as a premenstrual symptom?

As previously mentioned, despite being a widely recognised phenomenon, Premenstrual Syndrome (PMS) remains difficult to clinically define, with no universally agreed diagnostic criteria or shortlist of deterministic symptoms.[1] Indeed, the latest biomedical consensus is that 'any' symptoms count, so long as they occur in the two weeks prior to menstruation and are severe enough to limit normal daily tasks.[2] This lack of standardisation in definitions of PMS has contributed to a history of non-replicable and contradictory clinical research findings.[3]

The prevalence of PMS is similarly difficult to determine because without clear diagnostic boundaries, it is difficult to differentiate healthy premenstrual *changes* from problematic, sometimes debilitating, premenstrual *symptoms* requiring treatment.[4] As a result, population studies have variously claimed that PMS affects anything from 2.4 per cent[5] to over 80 per cent[6] of those who menstruate. Such wide-ranging claims call into question the validity of PMS as a diagnosis, since an illness that may affect 'hardly any' to 'nearly all' of such a large population is clearly prone to a high level of subjective interpretation.[7]

As you now know, PMS also exists as a highly gendered and stigmatised social label. Thus, critical scholars have persuasively argued that PMS is a socially constructed diagnosis that reflects the medicalisation of the female reproductive body – a process by which healthy changes are positioned as pathological and used to justify discriminatory beliefs and practices.[8] Biomedical descriptions of PMS are further critiqued for tending to position women's experiences of emotional distress as wholly or primarily biological in origin, rather than a rational human response to *distressing* embodied, psychological or social experiences.[9]

As a result, biomedical and critical PMS literatures are typically positioned as oppositional, incompatible and contradictory perspectives, creating two separate research streams.[10] However, both sides agree that premenstrual experiences are *biopsychosocial* phenomenon, meaning that there are biological, psychological and social factors involved. This chapter, therefore, begins with an overview of some identified biopsychosocial factors in premenstrual distress, beyond 'hormonal' explanations. The rest of the chapter describes how my research aims to integrate biological and psychosocial perspectives (and data), to more scientifically define 'what counts as a premenstrual symptom', without unintentionally pathologising the menstrual cycle or an entire gender.

Biopsychosocial factors in PMS

Despite positioning the biomedical label of PMS as socially constructed, critical scholars have always been aware that many women are happy to describe themselves as suffering from it, especially if this enables recognition of their experiences and access to support.[11] Critical scholars have, thus, set out to understand more about women's premenstrual experiences, and how and why they might describe them as PMS. As a result, this literature has identified several psychosocial factors that contribute to experiences and descriptions of premenstrual distress. These psychosocial factors have been grouped into two main themes: 'the concept of PMS as priming' and 'PMS as embodied psychosocial stress'.

The concept of PMS as priming

Studying the menstrual cycle is expensive and labour-intensive because it lasts an average of 28 days and to establish symptom cyclicity, data from at least two cycles (but ideally three) is required. This meant that the first biomedical PMS studies were all 'retrospective', simply asking women to recall their experiences over the past few cycles. Critical research has now consistently shown that this process is subject to various biases. The most obvious limitation being that it is extremely difficult for anyone to accurately retrieve memories of their experiences over a two- or three-month period.[12] More surprisingly, though, was the finding that the categories listed on questionnaires could influence an individual's recollection of the type, severity and frequency of premenstrual symptoms experienced.

   In one classic study by Diane Ruble, participants were randomly told that they were either 'premenstrual' or 'intermenstrual', or not told anything about their menstrual phase, even though they were all tested about a week before menstruation.[13] Those that had been assigned 'premenstrual' status were statistically more likely to report moderate to severe symptoms than either the 'intermenstrual' or control group.[14] This suggested that 'learned associations or beliefs might lead [an individual] either to overstate what [they] are actually experiencing or perceive an exaggeration of naturally fluctuating bodily states when [they] believe [they] are premenstrual'.[15] Similarly, clinical tracking tools based on the diagnostic criteria for Premenstrual Dysphoric Disorder (PMDD) appear to have primed people from cultures previously unlikely to associate mood changes with the menstrual cycle to start reporting them.[16]

As mentioned in Chapter 2, cultural norms and beliefs regarding menstruation are known to influence premenstrual experiences, with several studies finding that they appear to affect symptom perception, frequency and severity.[17] Individuals who described periods as a type of 'illness' were found to experience more frequent and severe premenstrual distress.[18] Similar results have been found by Maria Marvan and colleagues, when comparing the experiences of individuals exposed to a video about PMS as a negative phenomenon, with those who watched a more neutral video about the menstrual cycle. The negatively primed participants reported significantly more severe symptoms than the control group.[19] Correspondingly, when individuals were primed to associate the menstrual cycle with positive experiences, they reported fewer premenstrual symptoms.[20]

Interestingly, recent research has found that women self-identifying as 'PMS sufferers' may do so in a positive way, as a means to legitimise expressions of anger or low mood.[21] This suggests that societal/clinical disbelief in female-prevalent symptoms (and women's accounts of their experiences in general) is internalised, causing individuals to question the legitimacy of their own experiences, and so attribute them to PMS and the body rather than external stressors because biological causes are felt to be less *questionable*.

PMS as embodied interpersonal stress

Critical scholarship, especially the work of Jane Ussher and Janette Perz, has also argued that Western models of idealised *femininity* create an impossible standard (constant calmness, productivity, attractiveness and cheerfulness) to which women are supposed to, yet cannot, conform.[22] Irritability or temporary water retention, abdominal bloating or weight gain (often described as feeling 'out of control' or 'fat and ugly') are categorised as biomedical problems only when they occur in women.[23] Studies have shown that women may internalise these unrealistic standards and, thus, experience premenstrual distress in part due to *self-objectification* – a process by which an individual measures their behaviour and self-esteem against (idealised) societal discourses.[24] For instance, in women who identify as suffering from premenstrual disorders, symptom severity has been found to be associated with negative body image[25] and low body satisfaction.[26]

As well as existing in relation to societal discourses regarding femininity, premenstrual distress is also associated with more direct personal relationships mediated by gender norms. Several studies have identified 'relationship strain' as a key psychosocial factor in PMS and PMDD.[27] Indeed, (heterosexual) relationship satisfaction may decline just before menstruation.[28] It is also recognised that women who report PMS tend to self-silence and hide their emotions within relationships.[29] Correspondingly, more effective communication between couples has been found to reduce premenstrual distress,[30] especially if Cognitive Behavioural Therapy is directed at the couple (rather than just the individual).[31]

PMS studies involving lesbian couples (often in comparison to heterosexual ones) have found lower rates of reported premenstrual distress and that partners were more likely to provide non-judgemental support of experiences of premenstrual change.[32] Since other studies have previously identified an association between internalised 'idealised constructions of femininity' and premenstrual distress (the more feminine the more distress),[33] it could also be that lesbians are less likely to conform to idealised notions of femininity.[34] In short, research suggests that an individual's partner acts as a mediator of premenstrual distress, and that this relates to conformity to heterosexual gender roles and idealised femininity.[35]

Biological factors (beyond 'hormones')

Biomedical studies have also identified some biopsychosocial factors affecting those who report premenstrual distress. While the critical literature has tended to focus on the 'psychosocial' aspects, the biomedical literature has placed a little more emphasis on the 'biological' part. For instance, Warner and Bancroft (and colleagues) found that distress was significantly associated with increasing age/the number of consecutive periods an individual has had (without linking this to iron deficiency), previous diagnoses of mood disorders (including depression or anxiety), caring for young children, (heterosexual) cohabitation/marital status, unhappiness in romantic relationship, and part-time employment status (it was unclear if symptoms preceded part time work or vice versa).[36]

Logue and Moos found that people reporting PMS tended to have longer and heavier periods (without linking this to iron deficiency),[37] a history of mental illness and high levels of 'life stress'. Lee and Rittenhouse found that those diagnosed with a premenstrual disorder were more likely to have other physical and mental illnesses,[38] and less social support than the general menstruating population. There is also a known association between traumatic life experiences and the diagnosis of PMDD.[39] Finally, there is an association between smoking cigarettes and PMS, but it is not known if this is a coping mechanism or a causal factor.[40]

In summary, there is a body of scientific evidence regarding biopsychosocial factors in problematic cyclical experiences that is currently omitted from biomedical guidelines on PMS.[41] This is interesting because these findings are not directly contradicting or dismissing (hormonal) biological explanations. They provide useful information about the way in which widespread ignorance of menstrual health and associated gender myths, and the positioning of periods as stigmatising and inherently debilitating, can affect an individual's embodied premenstrual experiences. It is also not difficult to integrate psychosocial with biological causal theories, so this omission is not due to any sort of scientific complexity, or incompatible data issue.

One possible reason for the omission of psychosocial factors in clinical descriptions of PMS is the biomedical tendency to incorrectly position all critical work as 'political' (especially if feminist) and, thus, allegedly 'unscientific'.[42] Another compelling explanation was first put forward by Figert; the cyclic pattern in some individual's debilitating emotional distress seemed to provide a perfect example of 'biological' emotional distress.[43] When PMDD was first listed as a type of psychiatric disorder in 1987, a major shift was occurring within the discipline of psychiatry. This involved the rejection of psychoanalytic theories and practice (that is, counselling therapy for traumatic life experiences) in favour of (chemical) biological explanations and pharmaceutical treatments. It was hoped that this shift would provide more effective and efficient treatment options and boost the status and credibility of psychiatry.[44] Certainly, the biomedical PMS literature's subsequent omission of psychosocial research and its relentless (unsuccessful) quest to identify a hormonal cause of PMS seem to support Figert's hypothesis.

Similarly, the critical PMS literature has tended to ignore biology in favour of establishing psychosocial explanations for cyclical emotional distress. While it has always acknowledged a biological component in premenstrual experiences, the critical literature has typically been reluctant to actively engage with menstrual physiology, beyond pointing out that no hormonal causal mechanism has ever been proven. This could be because the bulk of the critical literature comes from critical health and social *psychology*, which as a discipline is highly sceptical of biological explanations for emotional distress. Certainly, explicitly *feminist* psychology has been reluctant to engage with biology because it has so often been used 'against women' in essentialist biological determinist justifications for the perpetuation of gender inequalities.[45] Unfortunately, this omission in the critical PMS literature has only reinforced claims that critical scholarship positions premenstrual experiences (as opposed to just their biomedical labels) as 'unreal' social constructs.[46]

The more recent critical work of Jane Ussher and Janette Perz has, therefore, tried to better integrate women's *embodied* experiences of physiological changes.[47] Ussher and Perz applied a *Critical Realist* approach to allow them 'to acknowledge the materiality of change across the menstrual cycle, including changes in [the body], mood, or women's perception of embodied change, but also to conceptualise this [experience] as mediated by culture, language, and politics'.[48] While the embodied 'biological' reality of cyclical changes was explicitly acknowledged in this work, however, analysis was still limited to patient *accounts of* associated distress, rather than integrating any biological data or explanations. Thus, prompting me to take the Critical Realist approach further in my doctoral study.

Comparing discourses to identify commonalities, differences and omissions

You should probably also know that before starting the PhD, I had already established that the symptoms most frequently cited in both the biomedical *and* critical PMS literatures were mood-based.[49] Given that population studies suggest that these are not the most common, uniquely determining or most disruptive premenstrual symptoms,[50] the scientific rationale for prioritising them over physical ones was unclear. In fact, I suspected that this arbitrary focus on emotional distress was most likely due to the (unintentional) influence of the myth of the hysterical/irrational/hormonal female.[51]

The main aim of my doctoral study was, therefore, to help better define and distinguish typically mild (healthy) premenstrual changes from debilitating (pathological) cyclic symptoms requiring medical/psychological/ social support. I planned to do this by comparing biomedical, critical and patient accounts of PMS, with robust data about the physiological origins, type, relative prevalence and severity of premenstrual symptoms in the general menstruating population. The rationale being that if not based on the available data, expert and lay descriptions of PMS *must* be influenced by other unscientific factors. I reasoned that by identifying and mitigating these factors, it might be possible to more accurately define and distinguish healthy versus pathological premenstrual experiences. Ultimately, I hoped that this approach could also help resolve some of the disputes that have arisen between critical and biomedical PMS scholarship, improve the quality of clinical research and practice, and better support those who experience debilitating cyclical symptoms, without (even unintentionally) stigmatising 'all women'.

I eventually settled on three interrelated research questions. My first and main research question was, 'How and why are certain premenstrual changes/symptoms prioritised over others in expert and patient descriptions of PMS?' If not based on the available empirical data, how do different stakeholders define what counts as a premenstrual symptom? What do their descriptions reveal about the influence of societal myths and assumptions within biomedical research? My second question, 'How do expert and patient descriptions of PMS compare with robust population data on premenstrual changes/symptoms?', examined 'whose accounts count' in PMS research and whose accounts are more in line with the available data. Finally, my third question, 'What are the possible implications of these expert and patient descriptions of premenstrual changes/symptoms?', sought to reveal the way in which PMS descriptions may (unintentionally) reproduce gender myths, be misinterpreted by others, or otherwise serve to obscure, medicalise or undermine *healthy* (pre)menstrual physiology and associated experiences.

Who did I interview?

To help you interpret and reflect on the findings discussed in the following chapters, I think it is useful to share some information about who was interviewed for the qualitative part of this study. All participants were selected using a purposive sampling approach.[52] Sampling in this way typically involves identifying individuals that are especially knowledgeable about (for example, PMS experts) or experienced with the research topic (for example, PMS patients).[53] Efforts were also made to purposefully select as diverse a group as possible within the parameters of the study. This was primarily to explore known factors in perspectives on PMS, such as certain embodied and material characteristics previously identified in the literature. For example, age,[54] sexuality and/or marital status,[55] socioeconomic status,[56] educational attainment,[57] ethnicity and/or cultural background,[58] and parity (whether you have had a child).[59]

Taking a purposeful approach avoided some of the limitations of sampling purely by *convenience*, which would have likely resulted in the recruitment of predominantly young, White, single, middle-class, heterosexual patients and far fewer, mainly male, UK-based PMS specialist gynaecologists through my existing academic and professional networks. Purposive sampling was thus important for two reasons: to enable a more nuanced qualitative analysis of participant interviews, and to include a more diverse range of patient perspectives and experiences than have typically been canvassed in qualitative PMS research to date, that is, young, White and middle-class women attending PMS clinics.[60]

The expert participants were all recruited via international professional networks. The patients were recruited through my existing personal and professional networks. In total, 28 people were interviewed: 13 biomedical experts, three critical experts and 12 self-identified PMS patients. Given that there are only around 35 biomedical and six critical PMS research experts in the world, getting to speak to almost half of them was fantastic! A short participant background survey was sent to everyone after I interviewed them (Appendix B). The anonymised group data is shown in Table 3.1.

Considering the small number of participants, diversity within the groups was very good across several characteristics. Some exceptions were: the sex of the expert participants (unfortunately, most of the biomedical experts who declined or failed to respond to the email invitation were male, leading to twice as many female than male participants); the age and employment status of the experts (predominantly close to or beyond retirement age, which is fairly representative of this group); the ethnicity of the experts (was entirely White, which is fairly representative of this group); and the high educational attainment level of the patients (all were university educated, or to a similar professional level).[61] Some unavoidable similarities related to

Table 3.1: Participant characteristics and information

	PMS experts (n=16)	PMS patients (n=12)
Sex (all cisgender)	12 female; 4 male	12 female
Age group	1 (25–34); 2 (45–54); 7 (55–64); 6 (65+)	7 (25–34); 4 (35–44)
Ethnicity (self-defined)	4 White British; 3 White European; 3 White Australian; 6 White North American	4 White British; 1 Mixed-race North American; 1 Punjabi North American; 3 Black British; 3 Bangladeshi British
Country of residence	4 UK; 6 USA/Canada; 3 Sweden; 3 Australia	10 UK; 2 USA/Canada
Childhood religion	2 prefer not to say; 7 Christian; 7 non-religious	3 Christian; 3 Islamic; 2 Jewish; 1 Sikh; 3 non-religious
Current religion	2 prefer not to say; 2 Christian; 2 Jewish; 10 non-religious	3 Christian; 1 Islamic; 1 Jewish; 1 Sikh; 6 non-religious
Number of children living at home	2 prefer not to say; 14 none	9 [none]; 2 [1 child]; 1 [2 children]
Marital status	2 prefer not to say; 13 married; 1 living with partner	1 married; 3 living with partner; 3 partner living elsewhere; 5 single
Sexuality	2 prefer not to say; 11 heterosexual; 3 homosexual	9 heterosexual; 3 bisexual
Highest educational qualification	2 prefer not to say; 7 postgraduate degree; 7 medical degree	1 professional qualification equivalent to degree level; 2 undergraduate degree; 8 postgraduate degree; 1 medical degree
Clinical/ academic discipline of qualification	2 clinical (other); 3 General Practice; 3 gynaecology; 3 psychiatry; 2 clinical psychology; 3 social psychology	3 non-health other; 4 health-related; 5 social sciences
Employment status	2 prefer not to say; 2 part-time employed; 8 full-time employed; 4 retired	1 student; 3 part-time employed; 8 full-time employed
Annual household income	7 prefer not to say; 9 (£80K+)	1 prefer not to say; 1 (under £20K); 3 (£20–29K); 1 (£30–39K); 2 (£50–59K); 2 (£60–69K); 2 (£80K+)
Affiliations	3 involved in creating the DSM definition of PMDD; 10 involved in creating other formal clinical definitions of PMS & PMDD; 4 members of the Society for Menstrual Cycle Research; 2 members of the International Association for Premenstrual Disorders; 3 members of the National Association for PMS (UK)	1 member of the Society for Menstrual Cycle Research; 1 member of the International Association for Premenstrual Disorders

the sex and age range of the patients, which reflects the temporary and sex-specific nature of the menstrual cycle. While I did reach out to a couple of transgender health networks, none of the trans men or non-binary people I met self-identified as suffering from PMS, either indicating that this was due to the suppression of their cycles with hormonal medications or simply not experiencing problematic cyclic changes. However, several people did mention period pain and the cyclical exacerbation of gender-dysmorphia as contributing reasons for suppressing their periods.

Separate expert and patient interview question lists were developed, based on their anticipated knowledge and experiences of PMS (Appendix C). Around half of the questions were the same in both lists to enable more straightforward comparison. The interviews were conducted according to participant preference and geographical limitations, either in person (n= 8), online video (n=18), by telephone (n=1) or email (n=1). The length of the expert interviews ranged from 21 to 83 minutes, with an average duration of 52 minutes. The interviews with patients ranged from 23 to 81 minutes, with a slightly longer average duration of 56 minutes. Two of the patients (Faith and Gemma) were interviewed at the same time (for their convenience) and one patient (Ria) was interviewed over two separate calls due to time constraints. Three of the experts (Fran, Celia and Laura) were asked a reduced selection of questions due to time constraints (only having half an hour in which to speak to me).

The audio recordings were transcribed as soon as possible after each interview, using an automated software. I then made manual corrections and notations to the text during repeated listening to the audio recordings (approximately four hours per interview). The software automatically identified and annotated the length of pauses and changes in speaker. Further annotation was added manually (Appendix D). For example, utterances such as 'um' or 'er', sighs, audible intakes or exhalations of breath, stuttering, extreme volume changes and emphasis on certain words were annotated using an adapted glossary of symbols, based on those first described by Jefferson (2004) (Appendix E). The interview transcripts were then anonymised before being uploaded to the qualitative data analysis software (NVivo) for further annotation and coding. This step was important because there are so few PMS experts in the world that without anonymisation, people might easily attribute the interview data to certain individuals.

Conducting Critical Realist Discourse Analysis

In line with the Critical Realist Discourse Analysis (CRDA) methodology outlined by Sims-Schouten and Riley, a 'three-level synthesised discourse analysis' was applied to the interview data.[62]

Step 1: Discursive Psychology analysis

First, a preliminary Discursive Psychology (DP) annotation and analysis of the data was carried out. DP approaches are more interested in what the talk is 'doing' than what the person is 'saying'. Seven discursive devices were found to be of most analytical value in this study; pronoun shifts (for example, from 'I' to 'we'); silences, pauses and hesitations; hedging talk (for example, repeated or stuttering speech or utterances of 'uh' or 'er'); minimisation (for example, language such as 'a bit', 'only' or 'just'); affect (for example, laughter, sighs or audible inhalation/exhalation); metaphor usage; and category entitlement labels (for example, 'women', 'psychiatrists' or 'gynaecologists').

For example, ten of the 16 expert participants displayed a distinct 'stuttering' speech pattern, typically when becoming aware of a possible contradiction in what they had just said. The following excerpt demonstrates the way in which this type of discursive 'disfluency' can sometimes signal a speaker trying to rapidly 'hedge' their words to absolve themselves of personal responsibility for the perceived inconsistency.[63] Also note the associated use of pronoun shifts between 'I' and 'they' (lines 1 to 3) to distance Andrew from the current American Psychiatric Association's Diagnostic and Statistical Manual of Mental Disorders (DSM) definition of PMDD (Excerpt 3.1).

Excerpt 3.1

1 I regard this as a kind of compromise [...] but still they do include them [typically
2 mild physical premenstrual changes in the diagnostic criteria for PMDD] (.) not
3 to annoy the gynaecologists too much (.) I assume (.) and I (.) if I (.) if I were king,
4 I would (.) I would have not regarded them as part of this at all [...] and I think
5 so (.) so (.) so (.) er (.) I (.) I (.) I believe that it's a (.) I think we should regard item
6 number eleven in the DSM as a compromise (.) and it's perhaps not that (.) er
7 (.) there's no robust scientific basis for that.
   (Andrew, biomedical expert)

Step 2: (Rhetorical) Discourse Analysis

Signs of discursive difficulty, such as these multiple or extended pauses, pronoun shifts, repetition and/or hedging talk, became highly *visible* during the process of DP annotation, which provided a valuable starting point for the second phase of Discourse Analysis (DA). Thus, after a transcript had been fully annotated according to the conventions of DP, I went back to the beginning and coded it again to provide an overall impression of the rhetorical content (that is, what people were talking about).

The purpose of this second analytical approach was to identify the ways in which the participants described their experiences of, or claims about, PMS.

The idea is that the 'discursive repertoire' of any given participant reflects their particular construction of 'what PMS is'. Inductive open coding was applied to discrete sentences and paragraphs, creating new or attributing existing codes to each discursive theme encountered in the data. Such coding is in line with Grounded Theory Methods, which derive meaning from data in a systematic way, as originally outlined by Glaser and Strauss.[64] The reason for using an exclusively inductive approach to the rhetorical coding was to minimise the influence of any preconceptions I had about any discursive themes I 'expected' to find in the data. All findings had to come *from* the data, I was not able to add any of my own knowledge or perspectives on PMS, beyond those conveyed by my choice of questions, and recorded verbal interactions with participants during the interviews.

The DA was initially carried out by hand on printed transcripts, before being organised into a hierarchical coding frame and transferred to a digital format using NVivo software. Initially, over 120 discourse codes were created, but during the digitisation process, these were refined and combined into 75 codes (Appendix F). Over five months of repeated and overlapping data collection and analysis, these codes were further refined into 42 *axial* codes, defined as 'aggregates of the most closely interrelated (or overlapping) open codes for which supporting evidence is strong' (Appendix F).[65] In turn, these axial codes were then grouped into the four major discursive themes described in detail over the following four chapters. Each theme is composed of roughly the same number of axial codes and associated excerpts of transcribed text.

Conducting repeated and combined DP and DA methods on each transcript, as well as across the gradually increasing dataset, provided unique and extremely valuable insights into the data. This approach enabled a more nuanced and empirically robust analysis of what, how and for what purpose discourses were being constructed by participants than would have been possible through DA alone. For example, by annotating all potential 'metaphors' (as part of DP), most of the participants were found to use of the concept of a 'normal curve' or 'spectrum of experiences' when describing PMS (Excerpt 3.2).

Excerpt 3.2

1   Um (.) like looking at the **normal curve and distribution** (.) a lot of PMS quote
2   unquote (.) [depicts quotation marks with hands] 'symptoms' (.) are just things
3   (.) ha! [laugh] (.) that happen to us during that time (.) which are like beautiful and
4   magical (pause) and also a huge struggle?
    (Ria, patient)

It was only by reflecting on the usage of the term 'normal' as a metaphor within specific contexts that one of the four main discursive themes (outlined in Chapter 5) evolved from being 'differentiating typically mild (that is, "normal" changes) from problematic premenstrual symptoms is difficult' (DA alone) to 'the use of the normal curve analogy enables debilitating cyclical symptoms (indicative of underlying health issues) to be positioned as simply a "more severe" version of typically mild premenstrual changes and vice versa' (DP plus DA). In short, it was possible to move beyond the identification of a recurring rhetorical trope in the data and gain valuable insight into *why* it may exist and *how* it is constructed through a particular discursive mechanism.

Step 3: Extra-discursive analysis

The third level of CRDA involved an analysis of the ways in which embodied, material or institutional factors may influence the participants' discursive repertoires.[66] The idea being that 'extra-discursive' contextual information (for example, the sex, cultural background, socioeconomic status or professional training) of an individual may 'provide the conditions of possibility that allows their sense-making to make sense'.[67] While the focus was on comparing expert with patient descriptions of PMS, these broad participant group categories were further disaggregated by various demographic characteristics established through the participant background survey: clinical/academic discipline, sex, age, ethnicity, sexual orientation, religious affiliation, nationality, marital status, parity/current childcare responsibilities, educational attainment and socioeconomic status (based on household income).

In practical terms, the interview data were split by question and participant group (experts and patients) in an Excel workbook. The discourses used by each participant were then compared within and across the participant groups. Around half of the participant questions allowed for direct comparison between the expert and patient groups, while the other half provided group-specific data. Discursive similarities and differences in the data were then identified and analysed with reference to the extra-discursive characteristics. This was to assess the level of discursive agreement within and between the participants across multiple intersecting embodied, material and institutional factors.

For example, the use of certain metaphors in participant descriptions of premenstrual experiences was found to vary between the expert and patient groups (Table 3.2).

In some instances, if an embodied/material/institutional factor was found to be of analytic relevance for a particular discourse, further comparative analysis was conducted using the NVivo software, especially regarding the frequency of specific terms or discursive device usage. For instance, when one of the patient-specific metaphors (dirty/toxic) was further analysed, it was found to be used *only* by patients with some sort of religious affiliation.

Table 3.2: The top ten metaphors used to describe premenstrual experiences and their relative usage by the expert and patient participants

Metaphor	# References	Approx. ratio of usage (experts: patients)
1. Normal curve/spectrum	131	4:3
2. Emotional	99	1:3
3. Hormonal imbalance	80	1:2
4. Crazy/irrational	63	1:4
5. Natural	58	1:4
6. Release/relief	52	1:8
7. Dirty/toxic	27	Only patients
8. Allergy/sensitivity	23	4:1
9. Out of control	12	1:1
10. Journey (of life)	11	Only patients

While qualitative research methods prohibit the generalisation of claims made about populations beyond the participants involved in the study, the identification of a potential relationship between a specific metaphor's usage and an extra-discursive factor such as religious affiliation could provide useful insight into its possible discursive *origins* and act as a prompt for future research. Not least because explicit descriptions of menstruation as an 'unclean' and spiritually, morally and physically 'impure' phenomenon are found within all the major religions' sacred texts and practices.[68]

Step 4: Data triangulation

Finally, wherever possible, the claims made in the interview data about 'what PMS is', what causes it and how prevalent it is within the population were compared with robust (quantitative) population data of relevance to these questions. Participant discourses were then ranked according to how closely they described the patterns identified in the population data. This step was in addition to the three typically implemented in CRDA.

In total, only four quantitative data sources were used to compare with the claims made by the interview participants (Table 3.3). They were selected based on their suitability (accessible raw data on symptom type, timing, prevalence and severity) and quality (large sample size, population sample method, geographical context, study inclusion criteria, data collection method, a measure of symptom severity included, and systematic reviews of multiple studies over single studies).

Table 3.3: The selection criteria for, and limitations of, the four datasets used to compare with the participant descriptions of PMS

Dataset	Participants	Rationale for selection	Main limitations
1. *The Epidemiology and Management of Premenstrual Symptoms in the community* (Mallia, 2015)	Prospective: Total n=7,742 Countries=5 Retrospective: Total n=33,065 Countries=18	Meta-analysis of 26 methodologically robust PMS population studies (8 prospective, 16 retrospective, 2 both). Theoretically robust and transparent study selection criteria and differentiation between retrospective and prospective studies. Large number of participants from 19 countries in total.	One of *only* two systematic reviews of this data in existence (although it is of good quality). It is an unpublished PhD thesis. The included studies typically lack control/comparative population data.
2. 'Global study of women's experiences of premenstrual symptoms and their effects on daily life' (Dennerstein et al, 2011)	Total n=7,226 Countries=11	A large-scale randomised study of women's experiences of premenstrual symptoms across 11 country contexts (including Asia). The *only* large-scale study with an open access dataset regarding reported symptom timing, prevalence, duration and debility.	Retrospective survey. The study provided a list of symptoms rather than inductively producing one from the data. Conducted in 2011, it is over a decade old. No control/comparative population data.
3. 'Mood and the menstrual cycle: A review of prospective data studies' (Romans et al, 2012)	Total n=4,279 Countries=10	A systematic review of the data from 47 studies on mood changes and the menstrual cycle. Prospective symptom data. Robust and transparent study selection criteria. Includes comparison data from non-menstruating participants. Reasonably large number of participants from ten countries.	It is the *only* systematic review of this data in existence (although it is of good quality). Conducted in 2012, it is over a decade old (although only a few additional prospective studies have since been published). Many studies provided a list of symptoms rather than inductively producing one from the data.
4. 'The association of inflammation with premenstrual symptoms' (Gold et al, 2016)	Total n=2,939 Ethnically diverse women from the United States	Reasonably large number of ethnically diverse participants, involved in a longitudinal population study. Data regarding several biomarkers collected and analysed. *Only* large-scale study to identify an association between physiological biomarkers and seven of the most common premenstrual symptoms (all of those assessed aside from headache).	Retrospective survey design, albeit randomised and using prospectively gathered biomarker data. Participants all based in the United States. Only eight of the most common premenstrual symptoms were assessed.

I started with Catriona Mallia's systematic review of PMS population studies since it is the most recent of only two such reviews ever conducted.[69] This provided robust quantitative data regarding the prevalence of premenstrual symptoms in general menstruating populations. I then read through all 26 studies included in Mallia's review and found that *only* Lorraine Dennerstein and colleague's cross-cultural epidemiological study had published the raw data regarding premenstrual symptom type, relative prevalence, duration and severity, along with comprehensive demographic information about the randomised sample population.[70] So, I selected it! Sarah Romans and colleagues' paper was included as the *only* systematic review of prospective studies on the timing and prevalence of mood-related symptoms in menstruating populations.[71] Finally, the Gold and colleagues' study was included as the *only* large-scale randomised and ethnically diverse population study that has identified a statistically significant association between some form of biomarker (inflammation markers) and premenstrual symptoms.[72]

As always, and especially because these data sources were often the 'only' robust large-scale quantitative data available, they were also subject to various limitations (outlined in Table 3.3). Overall, however, I was satisfied that the quality of data provided was sufficient for the purposes of this study.

A note on excerpts versus quotes and their labelling

Excerpts are used when elements of DP enabled a more insightful analysis of the interview data. For example, the use of metaphors, pronoun shifts or silences/hesitations. As a result, excerpt quotes are formatted according to the conventions associated with DP (Appendix D). For example, (.) denotes a short pause in speech. In contrast, participant *quotes* that are primarily of rhetorical 'thematic' value are shared without transcription annotation.

Bracketed labels such as (E2) or (P13) refer to the expert and patient question numbers associated with the described data (Appendix C). This is to promote transparency by helping readers to locate relevant content within the free to access dataset, available online.[73]

The following four chapters deal with the main themes identified in the interview data. As you will see, the influence of gender (and racial) myths on the expert and patient descriptions of PMS came out really clearly. See what you make of my findings, do you agree with my interpretation of the data? What do you think about the methodology? I am more than happy to be challenged on any element of this study. You can access the original interview data to read the interview transcripts and even conduct your own analyses.[75]

Box 3.1: What counts as a premenstrual symptom? Why this matters

Science

You may have spotted that all I was trying to do in this study was to implement a more scientific approach to the definition of premenstrual experiences. After all, ensuring that theories are based on the available empirical data, rather than opinions or conjecture, is a basic tenet of all scientific work. I simply could not understand why the biomedical PMS literature dismissed well-evidenced psychosocial factors in cyclical distress and the way in which gender stereotypes clearly influence, and are reproduced by, the diagnosis of PMS. Likewise, I was frustrated at how the critical PMS literature never got into the biology or epidemiology of cyclical experiences, beyond critiquing the inadequate 'hormonal' causal explanations provided by their biomedical 'opponents'. Why were these two research streams always portrayed as oppositional, anyway? This did not make any sense for a phenomenon that everyone apparently agrees is *biopsychosocial* in essence.

I was also aware that change does not happen easily if people are made to feel defensive, and thus more likely to cling on to their existing viewpoints. I hoped that by maintaining a neutral theoretical and disciplinary position, and anonymising the data, I could perhaps entice all sides of this definitional dilemma to engage with my work, without their risking any personal criticism. Another of the tenets of scientific enquiry is to embrace (evidence-based) criticism, but I think we all know that this is much easier said than done. Certainly, in the history of PMS research, we have around 40 years' worth of critical scholarship dismissed and omitted from most biomedical studies. Not to mention a century of ignoring or denying negative research findings regarding cyclic symptoms and the female sex hormones. This is why I also hoped that by revealing these and any other unscientific factors in current PMS research, it might be possible to avoid them in the future.

Integrating critical and biomedical scholarship on PMS is entirely possible, since this is what I do in my head all the time. This is partly why I suspected that the factors preventing integration must be political rather than scientific. I felt similarly about differentiating healthy from pathological cyclic experiences. My knowledge of healthy menstrual physiology (beyond its hormonal coordination) meant that I felt confident it was possible to differentiate typical (inflammatory) changes from more severe cyclic symptoms, usually indicative of underlying health conditions. This is not particularly complex or difficult science. It is simply allowing theories to be guided by the available physiological and population data.

Lastly, in terms of clinical research, having more robust definitions of cyclical symptoms (differentiated from healthy premenstrual changes) would help improve the quality of research into their possible causes, treatment options and prevalence in the population.

Clinical practice

Being better able to distinguish healthy from pathological cyclic changes is also important in terms of health outcomes and clinical interactions. Not only could more evidence-based definitions of cyclical health issues improve their diagnosis and treatment, but it would likely reduce the likelihood of patients being dismissed simply based on their gender and/or ethnicity.

Society

Just imagine if we could finally manage to disentangle gender (and racial) myths from biomedical and popular discourses about menstrual health, and other female-prevalent symptoms and conditions. We might no longer be subject to societal disbelief in, or minimisation of, our pain or other distressing life experiences. Female health research (beyond infertility) might even get funded! Female and/or racialised or otherwise marginalised leaders, colleagues, family members and victims of crime might no longer be treated as if 'hysterical' or inherently emotional/irrational. More realistically, it might at least reduce the number of times marginalised people have their opinions and experiences undermined by reference to their 'unbalanced' bodies or 'inferior psyches'? That would still be something.

Personal

It really would be great if we could finally unhitch female-prevalent symptoms, healthy menstrual changes and normal reactions to distressing or painful events from the myth of the hysterical/hormonal female. It could improve our health, wellbeing, self-esteem, earning potential and political status. Importantly, fewer of us (especially racialised women) might be forced to put up with chronic pain for much of our lives, or even risk dying in childbirth, simply because our words and expressions of pain and distress might be taken more seriously by those around us.[74]

4

Mind over matter: the psychologisation of premenstrual changes

This is the first of four chapters presenting the main themes of the interview data. This chapter focuses on the way in which some of the participant descriptions of Premenstrual Syndrome (PMS) revealed a tendency to position premenstrual changes as *psychological* rather than *physical* phenomena.

The first part focuses on how and why the expert participants separated and prioritised emotional distress, given that the patients described a mix of predominantly physical changes, in line with the available data. The second section examines the possible influence of the PMS stereotype in the positioning of premenstrual changes as more psychological than physical in origin, as well as experience. The third section argues that the way in which PMS was positioned in relation to Premenstrual Dysphoric Disorder (PMDD) was informed by and reproduces the PMS gender stereotype. The concluding section summarises the participant discourses and describes their possible implications.

The expert prioritisation of emotional distress

Early in the interviews, all participants were asked how they would describe PMS to someone who had never heard of it before. Interestingly, the expert descriptions of PMS differed from those of the patients *and* varied by clinical/ academic disciplinary affiliation. In fact, three distinct participant group definitions of PMS were consistently used throughout the interview data. These are referred to, from now on, as the 'biomedical expert' group, the 'critical expert' group, and the 'patient' group.

Biomedical PMS

Nine out of 13 biomedical experts described PMS as moderate to severe negative mood changes, only (or mainly).

> The cyclic occurrence of mood symptoms just before menses. (Barbara, biomedical expert [E2])

> I describe it as a sense of overwhelming tension … frequently accompanied by irritability and dysphoria (sort of a mixture of

irritability, depression and anxiety) occurring typically in the few days prior to the onset of menses and then continuing often into the menstrual period for a day or two. (Laura, biomedical expert [E2])

For most of the biomedical experts to describe PMS in this way was extremely surprising. Seven of these nine individuals were involved in the development of the formal biomedical definition of PMS, which clearly states that 'it is the timing, rather than the types of symptoms, and the degree of impact on daily activity that supports a diagnosis of PMS. The character of symptoms in an individual patient does not influence the diagnosis'.[1]

Framing PMS as a moderate to severe mood-based phenomenon risks confusing it with PMDD, a supposedly discrete diagnostic category. In fact, while describing PMS, four of the biomedical experts mentioned suicidal ideation, something that is formally associated with PMDD, or the premenstrual exacerbation (PME) of underlying mental health conditions, such as depression and anxiety. 'It's [PMS] a mood disorder which occurs only premenstrually … and the symptoms … can be so bad as to promote suicidal ideation or attempt' (Chris, biomedical expert [E2]).

The association with suicidal ideation may partly explain the biomedical experts' prioritisation of premenstrual mood changes. Severe mental health crises of this sort are far more life-threatening than other types of premenstrual change. For clinicians, morally, institutionally and sometimes legally responsible for the health and wellbeing of patients, any disclosure of suicidal ideation is, thus, justifiably prioritised. Three of the biomedical experts plainly described the relative urgency and subsequent prioritisation of this behaviour during their interviews. Chris went on to describe how suicidal ideation was considered more 'important' than other premenstrual symptoms, even though it was an uncommon occurrence: 'There is also the question of how common they [premenstrual symptoms] are and how important they are, 'cos suicidal ideation is obviously less common, but more important than anxiety' (Chris, biomedical expert [E10]).

Sarah even suggested that PMS/PMDD clinical specialists (especially 'psychiatrists' in line 1) only saw patients with acute mental health symptoms, since physical premenstrual symptoms were more easily dealt with by a *non-PMS-specialist* 'gynaecologist or GP' (line 3) (Excerpt 4.1). The framing of suicidal ideation as a 'real issue' in comparison to more common premenstrual experiences (line 6) also supported the idea that mood changes were *disproportionately* prioritised due to the risk of death or serious injury.

Excerpt 4.1

1 [U]m (.) but for the psychiatrists (.) ha! [laugh] of course (.) that's
2 [mood changes] what they're most concerned about (.) it's not women coming with (.)
3 heh! [laugh] mastalgia (.) they're going to go to their gynaecologist or a GP (.) but (.)
4 but you know (.) they're gonna be referred the woman with the really problematic
5 depression who may be suicidal at that time (.) um (.) you know (.) that becomes
6 a real issue.
   (Sarah, biomedical expert [E11])

Critical PMS

In contrast to the biomedical experts, the critical expert accounts of PMS placed greater emphasis on an individual's external context: 'That week or so before um, a woman's period where she is more sensitive and more vulnerable um, to um, changes both within her body but also externally to stimuli and to environmental, um, stressors' (Zoe, critical expert [E2]). This group also prioritised emotional distress but described it as triggered *in response* to life experiences and physical premenstrual changes, rather than physiologically induced negative mood changes, as such. Thus, while all the PMS experts prioritised the same type of premenstrual experience (emotional distress), their accounts revealed an important difference between critical and biomedical disciplines in their object of study and its causal mechanism. In crude terms, the critical experts emphasised external psychosocial factors, while the biomedical experts emphasised internal biological factors, in what both groups apparently agreed was a mood-based biopsychosocial phenomenon.

This suggested that the critical experts' focus on emotional distress over other types of premenstrual change was mainly due to their contestation of purely, or predominantly, biological explanations for women's emotional distress. Especially since these explanations imply that the healthy female body is the primary cause of emotional distress, rather than it being a reasonable response to *distressing* life circumstances. The critical experts did not, however, explicitly contest the disproportionate prioritisation of this type of experience over physical ones.

Patient PMS

Finally, the patient group typically described PMS as referring to 'all premenstrual changes' (physical, behavioural and mood-related), ranging from very mild to debilitating.

Feeling just tired or a bit down and you don't know why and you're more likely to cry at things. But it, it can also mean that you get a bit of an upset tummy or, well, you find it a bit hard to go for a poo. (Beth, patient [P13])

A collection of symptoms that vary from person to person with a period (pause) you know, it could be anything from mild irritability and weeping all the way to severe cramping, you know, exhaustion. (Helen, patient [P13])

Crucially, the patient group's descriptions of PMS most closely resembled robust population data on the type and relative frequency of the most common premenstrual symptoms.[2] The patients did not, however, tend to differentiate between debilitating and typically mild premenstrual experiences.

Interestingly, the differences in expert and patient participant group definitions were also apparent when comparing the type and number of symptoms they described. When asked to list the 'most common' premenstrual symptoms, the biomedical experts listed about twice as many mood symptoms than physical symptoms on average (Table 4.1). The critical experts mentioned equal numbers of mood and physical symptoms, and the patients typically described about twice as many physical than mood symptoms (Table 4.1). Again, it was the patient group's description (an approximate ratio of mood: physical symptoms of 1:2) that was closest to the findings of the large-scale study of premenstrual symptoms conducted by Dennerstein and colleagues.[3]

Premenstrual changes as 'all in her mind'

Beyond the three participant group definitions of PMS lay another highly accessible discourse, the PMS stereotype. Crucially, descriptions of this stereotype were remarkably consistent across the participant groups. When

Table 4.1: What are the most common premenstrual symptoms? Average number and type of symptoms mentioned by participant group

	Mood	Behavioural	Physical	Total	Approximate ratio mood: physical
Biomedical experts (n=13)	3.7	1.2	1.8	6.6	2:1
Critical experts (n=3)	3.3	1.3	3.3	8.0	1:1
Patients (n=12)	1.4	1.3	3.2	5.8	1:2
Population data (top 10 changes) (Dennerstein et al, 2011) (n=7,226)	3	1	6	10	1:2

asked if they had heard of a PMS stereotype, only one patient said that they had not, and three of the biomedical experts admitted they had heard of one but did not describe it. The remaining 24 participants universally portrayed an 'irrational' and pathologically 'emotional' (typically 'irritable' but sometimes also 'sad') woman.

> The sort of mad, bad, and dangerous, really. That a woman is irrational and out of control, violent, crazy. Not to be taken seriously. (Susan, critical expert [E8])

> A woman being out of control, or completely full of rage, or bawling her eyes out, or an emotional wreck. (Emma, patient [P19])

The stereotype was highly gendered, with nearly all participants describing it as applicable to 'all women' regardless of their reproductive status or experiences. Five participants also added qualifiers of consensus, such as 'of course', to suggest that this stereotype was extremely well known and established over time. Indeed, the stereotype described by the participants appeared to be a contemporary iteration of the hysteria gender myth.

> That would be women, angry women, of course. (Marta, biomedical expert [E8])

> Yeah, of course, there's like the moody, angry, irrational woman. (Dani, patient [P19])

Disbelief in (racialised) patient experiences

While most of the participants appeared to dismiss the validity of the PMS stereotype, it clearly still influenced the way in which they experienced and/or engaged with PMS as a biomedical label. For instance, during the interviews, several of the participants implied that the PMS stereotype positioned premenstrual changes as 'unreal', 'imagined', 'exaggerated' or 'psychological' in origin. Anne described how some of the visitors to a public exhibition about PMS reacted as if the term was simply a contrived 'excuse' for irritability or anger (when expressed by women): 'The other group of people either didn't know about it [PMS], or almost (pause) erm (pause) used it as a, as though it's "women making an excuse to be irritable or angry"' (Anne, biomedical expert [E8]).

This aspect of the PMS stereotype and associated gender myths encourages others' dismissal of, or disbelief in, the legitimacy of women's experiences and perspectives. In fact, when asked why PMS might be considered a controversial diagnosis, 'disbelief' was the most common patient response,

Figure 4.1: Top ten responses to 'PMS is considered by some to be a controversial diagnosis, what is your understanding of why this might be?'

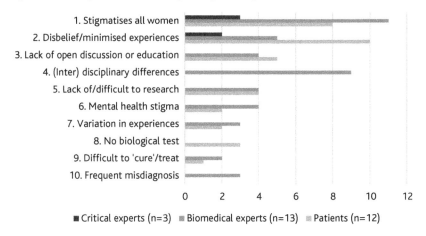

closely followed by 'it stigmatises all women' (Figure 4.1). A quarter of the patients also mentioned the lack of any objective medical test for PMS, implying that without tangible *proof*, women's reporting of premenstrual symptoms is inherently questionable (number 8 in Figure 4.1).

When asked a follow-up question about their experiences of others' disbelief in their premenstrual symptoms, over half of the patients described specific encounters with partners, family members, peers, teachers, colleagues or general practitioners (GPs). Helen's response illustrated the way in which her partner's disbelief (expressed through 'reported speech') was clearly informed by the PMS stereotype ('you're just being irrational' and 'you're being overemotional' in lines 3 and 4) and how it overlapped with mental health stigma (line 2), implying a conceptual link between premenstrual changes and mental health disorders (Excerpt 4.2).

Excerpt 4.2

1 [H]e thought I was just being weak minded (.) like he absolutely subscribed
2 to the general view of all things premenstrually or mental health-related (.) as 'you
3 can think your way out of this' (.) 'you can't be as bad as you say' (.) 'you're just being
4 irrational' (.) 'you're being overemotional' (.) I think that was (.) to this day (.) the
5 hardest one to swallow (pause) is the lack of believing from my own partner.
   (Helen, patient [P29])

Only five of the 12 patients stated that they had ever consulted a doctor about PMS, and several patients implied that they did not trust doctors to take their experiences seriously. In fact, of those who did seek professional help for their premenstrual symptoms, four out of five described how their doctors either directly dismissed, failed to diagnose or did not offer an effective treatment. Helen mentioned how her severe pelvic pain and mood symptoms (eventually diagnosed as fibroids and PMDD) were initially positioned as entirely psychological in origin, a dismissal seemingly due to her gender, as also reflected by the strikingly stereotypical treatment recommendation, 'go shopping': 'I mean, I was told "this is all in your head" … I was never given like a consistent, straight thing outside of "Go home, take a Midol, go shopping, you'll feel better"' (Helen, patient [P17]).

The small number of participants prevents generalisation, but the data suggested that some patients were perhaps more likely to have experienced disbelief in their premenstrual symptoms than others. Five out of seven of the Black British, Bangladeshi British or mixed-race US patients described members of their close family as sceptical of their experiences, and three of them attributed this to 'cultural' reasons.

> Oh my gosh! It's such a hard thing to navigate when your family are African [laugh]. I mean, 'this is the way of life, you must, this is normal, like what's your problem? We've all done it before'. (Gemma, patient [P7])

> Yeah, I think in my community, I think it's because we come from, um, I come from an Asian community. We do dismiss a lot of things … it's seen as an excuse to get out of things … or just excuse for the way you're acting. (Mala, patient [P29])

In contrast, none of the four White British patients described a similar experience. This pattern is in line with studies that have found cultural differences in illness perceptions and pain beliefs.[4] It also seems to support Chrisler's concept of PMS as predominantly (or at least, originally) a White North American/Western European 'culture-bound' gender construct.[5]

Also, all but one of the Black and ethnic minority patients described experiencing disbelief in/dismissal of their premenstrual experiences from managers or work colleagues, teachers or doctors, in contrast with only one of the White patients. This finding is in line with several studies that have found Black and other racialised ethnic minority women are more likely to be pejoratively stereotyped as inherently 'angry'[6] or 'tolerant of pain',[7] contributing to a higher likelihood of being disbelieved and dismissed by others.[8] A couple of the patients seemed aware of these issues, in fact, Gemma explicitly stated that she did not trust doctors to take her experiences (as a Black woman) seriously: 'So, it's because like they have, because they kind of internalise that you can handle the pain. … I've had really negative experiences with doctors. I don't go to the doctors … they would never sit me down and examine me' (Gemma, patient [P17]).

Critical perspectives and the PMS stereotype

The PMS stereotype also appears to have had an impact on the experiences and perspectives of the critical experts. During the interviews, social constructionist approaches, such as those used by the critical experts, were directly referenced by two of the patients and two biomedical experts. All four positioned this work as contributing to societal disbelief in severe premenstrual symptoms.

> I had a discussion with this person who, who (pause) was questioning whether or not we have been socialised into believing that PMS is a, is a cult-, is a socially constructed thing, and it's not a biological thing. And that was really difficult to hear. Yeah, so yeah. I've come across people who don't believe in it or don't believe it's a thing and don't understand how it can affect people. (Emma, patient [P29])

Unsurprisingly, the three critical experts who use social constructionist approaches in their work insisted that they did not dismiss or invalidate the experiences of those with severe cyclical symptoms. They described their position as simply contesting the unnecessary medicalisation of non-pathological premenstrual changes, and the attribution of emotional distress entirely to the female reproductive body (that is, their explicit purpose was to contest the PMS stereotype and associated gender myths). 'My interest has been in this stereotype notion that all women have the same experience, that all women go crazy right before their period, which is not true. But that's not to say that no women suffer' (Geraldine, critical expert [E17]).

In short, a somewhat ironic situation arose in that the critical experts' valid contestation of the PMS stereotype (most women do not experience problematic premenstrual changes and cyclical distress is not *only* biological in origin) was misinterpreted by others as reinforcing another aspect of it (premenstrual changes are 'all in her mind') and, thus, was itself subject to disbelief. This undermines the work of the critical academics who, in their efforts to counter negative gender myths, were accused of invalidating the experiences of some women. Significantly, it appeared that the fact that the critical experts were talking about a psychosocial rather than biological phenomenon was not obvious because the same term (PMS) was used to describe the same type of experience (emotional distress).

Biomedical perspectives and the PMS stereotype

The biomedical experts also appeared to be influenced by the PMS stereotype. In addition to their disproportionate prioritisation of moderate to severe mood-related changes, they tended to position PMS as a type of 'mental health disorder', sometimes explicitly: 'I would describe it [PMS] as a menstrual mental health condition' (Anne, biomedical expert [E2]). More often, the biomedical experts did so by comparing PMS to 'other' mental health conditions. The following excerpt illustrates the way in which the comparison between PMS (as opposed to PMDD) and 'lots of mental health conditions' (line 1), such as ADHD (line 3) and depression (line 4), unintentionally perpetuated the stereotypical belief that premenstrual changes are predominantly psychological rather than physical, in origin (as well as experience) (Excerpt 4.3).

Excerpt 4.3

1   I think there's a general misunderstanding of lots of mental health
2   conditions (.) and I don't think this [PMS] is peculiar in that regard (.) so I treat adults
3   with ADHD as an example (.) and there's still a debate going on as to whether ADHD
4   really exists (.) some people will say the same thing about general depression (.) that
5   doesn't exist and people should just pull their socks up [audible exhale] (pause) so I
6   don't think it's peculiar to (.) to PMS [...] anything that involves the mind (.) leads
7   some people to believe that you should be able to control it yourself.
    (John, biomedical expert [E17])

An obvious difference between other mental health conditions and premenstrual negative mood changes, however, is that their regular cyclical occurrence *demands* some sort of physiological explanation, even if they are simultaneously positioned as 'all in the mind'. This creates a contradiction within stereotypical and biomedical descriptions of PMS, potentially contributing to societal disbelief in the premenstrual experiences of women, as eloquently described by Helen, one of the patients.

> I think it's funny, I feel like society attributes 'like we yeah, we get this is part of your biology, your body's like doing its thang, but we also think you're being weak minded at the same time, like get over it!' You know what I mean? It's like 'we're going to pretend it's all, it's equally there and not there. That it's out of your control, but also in your control' [laugh]. (Helen, patient [P19])

This paradox was also reflected in the way that two-thirds of the biomedical experts implied that typically mild and non-pathological premenstrual changes such as temporary breast swelling or weight gain were part of PMDD (a psychiatric disorder). In contrast, the critical experts maintained that such changes had no place in the diagnostic criteria for PMDD. It was, therefore, the biomedical, rather than the critical social constructionist, discourse that positioned typical premenstrual changes as being part of a mental health disorder, thus implying they were perhaps psychological in origin. A particularly revealing example of this logical inversion is found in two of the biomedical experts' responses to this question. They seemed to imply that physical premenstrual changes could even be *caused* by PMDD (a psychiatric disorder).

> Many if not all mental diagnoses have physical symptoms. Anxiety is one example of a mental issue that manifests in many physical symptoms. (Barbara, biomedical expert [E22])

> If you do look at studies or you ask patients who have depression, most of them have pain. In fact, it's very common to have pain, physical pain. And so, to say that it doesn't belong in a mental health diagnosis, I think isn't true. (Celia, biomedical expert [E22])

These quotes illustrate how the biomedical experts' prioritisation of moderate to severe premenstrual mood symptoms seemed to restrict their engagement with far more common physical changes and healthy menstrual physiology. This partial perspective was (unintentionally) influenced by, and reproduced, the PMS stereotype, by implying that premenstrual changes were mainly psychological in origin, as well as experience.

Much ado about PMDD

Finally, all participants were asked if they had heard of PMDD, and if so, to describe how it differed from PMS. Starting with the biomedical experts, around half of the group positioned PMS as essentially the 'same thing' as PMDD, only differing in symptom severity: 'I think some people say PMS and mean PMDD, and some people mean mild, some people say mild PMDD and they mean PMS. I don't think that they're functionally different things' (Debbie, biomedical expert [E11]). In fact, one biomedical expert positioned the two labels as simply different terms by which biomedical experts in the United States and the United Kingdom refer to *exactly the same* experiences: 'I think that's just um (pause) a UK/ States thing. I don't think they're any different. I think it's just um, how it's been identified in different countries' (Jo, biomedical expert [E11]).

Again, this conflation of the terms PMS and PMDD is very surprising, given that several members of the biomedical expert group were directly involved in the development of the formal biomedical definitions of both, ostensibly distinct, diagnostic categories: one gynaecological,[9] the other psychiatric.[10] One biomedical expert even explicitly referenced these different formal definitions but stated they were mainly for 'scientific purposes' (that is, clinical research rather than clinical practice). For her, too, the only difference in terms of patient experience was symptom severity: 'I see PMS as a milder condition … that's, that's just the way I see it. … We have the different criteria for scientific purposes but if you ask me how I see it, I think it's a matter of severity' (Marta, biomedical expert [E11]).

The biomedical positioning of PMDD

Revealingly, the PMDD as 'severe PMS' analogy seemed to work both ways for some of the biomedical experts. When asked, around two-thirds of the group implied that they were happy with the endorsement of PMDD-specific daily symptom rating tools in the diagnostic guidelines for PMS. Five of these biomedical experts went on to imply that this was entirely appropriate because PMS is essentially 'less severe PMDD': 'Well there aren't other criteria for PMS and most people feel that PMS is a less severe form than PMDD. Maybe not quite five symptoms, maybe just lasting a couple of days, maybe less severe symptoms?' (Fran, biomedical expert [E19]).

As well as conflating two supposedly distinct biomedical diagnostic labels, this position is not in line with the available population data. For instance, Sarah Romans and colleagues' systematic review of 47 prospective studies on mood and the menstrual cycle found no evidence of a premenstrual negative mood pattern in the general menstruating population.[11] This suggests that the severe negative mood changes (including suicidal ideation) associated with PMDD cannot simply be described as a 'more severe version' of typical premenstrual changes. In fact, the data suggest that PMDD is far more likely to be the exacerbation of underlying emotional distress/mental health conditions.

The other half of the biomedical expert group who did not imply that PMDD was 'severe PMS' positioned it as a '*subcategory*' of PMS, instead: 'So, impairment is much greater with PMDD than PMS, but PMS is kind of, or PMDD is a subset, if you will, of PMS. So, there's this larger group with PMS and then there's this subset of people who have emotional symptoms, and it's really impairing, you know' (Laura, biomedical expert [E11]). The subcategory analogy is a little more consistent with the available data than the 'severe PMS' one, since it allows PMDD to be categorised as a debilitating premenstrual mood disorder, within a wider population of people who experience premenstrual changes of various types. It did not, however, help to clarify the ambiguous diagnostic boundaries of PMS, except to imply that the label covered *any* symptoms that are problematic but do not strictly fulfil the current diagnostic criteria for PMDD. This position was at least in line with the current UK formal biomedical definition of PMS developed by several of the biomedical expert group.[12]

Positioning PMDD as a subcategory of PMS, however, also implies a different sort of relationship than that between PMS and the exacerbation of underlying mental or physical health conditions. Or, put simply, that PMDD and PMS are more similar to each other (in terms of causal mechanism and type of experience) than they are to cyclical symptoms categorised as PME (premenstrual exacerbation), such as those associated with catamenial epilepsy, menstrual migraine, cyclical asthma or even the cyclic worsening of chronic depression or anxiety.

Indeed, when asked if symptoms associated with the exacerbation of an underlying health condition counted as premenstrual symptoms, all but two of the biomedical experts stated, if not insisted, that they did not. In fact, the group seemed to make a clear categorical distinction between the exacerbation of underlying conditions and both PMS and PMDD. Yet, in answering the question, around half of them also described how difficult it was, in practical terms, to separate or distinguish the diagnosis of PMDD from the exacerbation of an underlying mental health condition. One of the biomedical experts' responses is worth quoting at length, since it demonstrated the somewhat arbitrary, and frequently overlapping, nature of these diagnostic 'boundaries' (lines 1 to 6), plus the role of the patient in deciding how to label their experiences (lines 6 to 9) (Excerpt 4.4).

Excerpt 4.4

1 It becomes very difficult actually (.) to decide whether somebody
2 has PMDD as strictly defined by DSM 5 or whether they do actually have an
3 exacerbation of something (.) and even if somebody doesn't think they have
4 an exacerbation of something (.) there's always a question mark as to
5 whether or not it's just below the level of their (.) errr (.) conscious or
6 unconscious um (.) recognition (.) but I would say that many of the people that
7 I see (.) when you drill down (.) even though they might not complain of those
8 symptoms during the first half of the cycle (.) will acknowledge that they're
9 there to some degree [...] and I think there probably is a pure form of PMDD
10 (.) but I also think there's probably a lot of people that have (.) something else
11 that's bubbling away (.) that's exacerbated premenstrually.
   (John, biomedical expert [E14])

This excerpt also highlights the way in which John was confident that a 'pure' form of PMDD existed (line 9), despite acknowledging that making an accurate differential diagnosis between this and the exacerbation of an underlying mental health disorder was difficult (lines 1 to 6) (Excerpt 4.4). The concept of a 'pure' premenstrual disorder demonstrates the positioning of negative mood as intrinsic to the biomedical experts' description of PMS in a way that other (more common) physical premenstrual changes were not.

Critical perspectives on PMDD

The critical experts 'quoted' the biomedical literature when asked about the difference(s) between PMS and PMDD. While it was clear they did not personally define cyclical emotional distress in precisely the same terms as these sources, they nevertheless referenced them when asked questions that were otherwise difficult to answer. As a result, two of the three critical experts also appeared to position PMDD as 'more severe PMS' and vice versa (in response to a question about the use of PMDD tools to diagnose PMS). They did so, however, in terms that made it clear that they found the comparison incompatible with their preferred social constructionist explanation for premenstrual emotional distress. For example, Susan used category entitlement terms ('researchers' and 'clinicians' in lines 1 and 4) and associated pronouns ('they'll' in line 1) to distance herself from the biomedical terminology, as well as explicitly describing them as 'social constructs' (lines 3 and 4) (Excerpt 4.5).

Excerpt 4.5

1 [I]n terms of what it (.) how menstrual cycle researchers tend to use it
2 is (.) they'll say women with severe symptoms have PMDD (.) as if it's a thing (.) and
3 women with moderate symptoms have PMS as if it's a thing (.) but they're both social
4 constructs (.) they are both diagnostic labels that are created by clinicians.
  (Susan, critical expert [E11])

Another critical expert went on to imply that the two biomedical terms are somewhat interchangeable, depending on the clinical discipline of the specialist.

> Well [exhale] the psychiatrists say that PPDD [*sic*] is more serious, but you know, a smart-alecky comment about it would just be 'who are you going to, to get some help?' So, if you're going to a psychiatrist, you're going to get a PMDD diagnosis. If you talk to your general practitioner or your OBGYN, you, you're going to get the PMS definition or diagnosis. (Geraldine, critical expert [E11])

In contrast, the remaining critical expert unequivocally differentiated PMS from PMDD. It was implied that the social constructionist explanation for premenstrual emotional distress could not fully account for the severe symptoms (such as suicidal ideation) associated with the PMDD diagnosis, and that this made it a categorically different experience. 'I think PMDD is different. I think PMDD is a different set of experiences to just severe PMS' (Zoe, critical expert [E17]). This made Zoe the only PMS expert to explicitly describe the relationship between the biomedical labels PMS and PMDD in terms that reflected the available data.[13] In short, that the type of severe mental health symptoms associated with PMDD were not simply a 'more severe' version of typical premenstrual changes. Interestingly, in response to a later question about the premenstrual exacerbation of underlying conditions, another of the critical experts also suggested that PMDD was perhaps more accurately described as the 'worsening' of chronic depression, and that this was a position that many feminist critics took when PMDD was first listed in the DSM.[14] 'That's one of the arguments that a lot of feminists made about putting PMDD into the psychiatric nomenclature, is that these women may be depressed. You know, need a diagnosis of depression, not PMDD, but their depression might be worse or more salient at certain points of the cycle' (Geraldine, critical expert [E14]). The relative lack of clinical attention on the Premenstrual Exacerbation (PME) of depression and/or anxiety (as opposed to PMS/PMDD) was mentioned by Susan in response to the same question.

> There's not a huge amount of research on this [PME], which I think is interesting. And I suppose what I would say is, if this was happening to men there would be masses of research and masses of funding on this because if you have a chronic condition and ... it gets worse once a month, that's a really pretty bad thing. And we need to understand why. (Susan, critical expert [E14])

It thus appeared that the critical experts were relatively more inclined than the biomedical experts to position the type of severe emotional distress associated with the diagnostic label of PMDD as a form of PME, rather than a 'more severe' version of PMS (in line with the population data).

Patient perspectives on PMDD

When asked, around half of the patients stated that they had never heard of PMDD. Similarly, their responses to a later question about the exacerbation of underlying health issues, such as migraine or epilepsy, indicated that this group was very unfamiliar with this term or concept (the only two exceptions were Beth, who is also a GP, and Emma, who runs a PMDD awareness-raising organisation). This suggested that these terms and concepts existed primarily as clinical and academic labels, and so, due to a lack of alternative terminology, the patients might be more likely to describe the same experiences as PMS. Indeed, this was explicitly stated by one patient: 'It is hard to say. It's like what is being, what is a premenstrual exacerbation? See it's like, I would file premenstrual exacerbation under PMS almost, you know?' (Helen, patient [P26]).

Interestingly, when asked about the difference(s) between PMS and PMDD, all seven of the patients who had heard of PMDD mentioned symptom severity, but only three described any sort of difference in symptom type. Describing PMDD as something akin to 'severe PMS' was also implied in all but one of the seven patient responses.

> I have [heard of PMDD] but not like in depth, just of that, the PMDD. (Pause) I don't know, but I think that one is more of the intense one? (Noor, patient [P20])

> Yeah, I've definitely heard of it [PMDD]. I think that it is a much more extreme version where like the person suffering from it can actually feel suicidal, and (pause) incredibly unstable and unhappy at certain times? (Dani, patient [P20])

While the positioning of PMDD as 'severe PMS' is very much in keeping with the biomedical experts' typical description of PMS (as moderate to severe mood changes), it seems to contradict the patient group's 'any and all premenstrual changes' definition. It is impossible to know for sure, but it could be that the patients switched to alternative (mood-based) definitions of PMS to allow this analogy to make logical sense.

Chapter summary

In terms of how and why certain premenstrual changes were prioritised over others, the expert and patient descriptions of PMS were extremely illuminating. While in line with previous research findings,[15] the biomedical experts' consistent accounts of severe negative mood changes were still surprising given that ten of them were directly involved in the formal 'any symptom counts' definition of PMS. This description also contradicts robust population data regarding the most common premenstrual symptoms as predominantly physical in nature.

A couple of factors were mentioned that may partly account for the experts' focus on mood. In particular, the urgent and serious threat to patient life and health posed by cyclical suicidal ideation, and the fact that physical premenstrual symptoms are more easily treated by non-specialist clinicians. However, the ways in which the biomedical experts tended to position PMS as a type of mental health disorder, and more closely associated with PMDD than with any other premenstrually exacerbated conditions, suggested that they were also (unintentionally) influenced by the PMS stereotype (a contemporary version of the myth of the hysterical female).

The critical experts also prioritised emotional distress but defined PMS as referring to an individual's *response* to various types of embodied premenstrual changes, informed by their psychosocial context. By using the same term to describe a slightly different thing, the critical experts' valid claims about the socially constructed nature of the PMS diagnostic label were misinterpreted by some patients and biomedical experts, as implying that severe cyclic symptoms were, in themselves, 'unreal'. In fact, their focus on psychosocial factors in emotional distress served to explicitly counter the PMS stereotype/gender myth, that is, the positioning of 'all women' as necessarily debilitated (and rendered irrational/emotional) by the female (reproductive) body. Indeed, the critical experts were the only participants to position severe cyclical negative mood changes (such as suicidal ideation) as the exacerbation of chronic emotional distress, rather than 'severe PMS', which is more in line with the available data. By prioritising emotional distress over more common physical experiences, however, the group did also (unintentionally) reproduce the stereotypical positioning of premenstrual changes as predominantly psychological in experience.

The patients' descriptions of PMS were the most in line with the available population data, in that they mentioned predominantly physical premenstrual changes, although they did not differentiate between mild changes and severe cyclic symptoms (discussed in Chapter 5). This is perhaps unsurprising given that the patients were talking about their own embodied experiences. Indeed, the patients explicitly described the way in which the PMS stereotype had negatively impacted their lives, especially regarding others' dismissal of, or disbelief in, their experiences. The group was relatively unfamiliar with the terms PMDD and PME, which suggested that these were less accessible descriptions of premenstrual change contained within biomedicine and academia. Of those patients who were aware of PMDD, nearly all positioned it as 'severe PMS', in line with the biomedical expert discourses. This could either indicate that these individuals were simply quoting biomedical discourse, and/or they switched to more stereotypical portrayals of PMS as predominantly mood-based, to allow the analogy to 'make sense'.

In short, several participant discourses were not based on the available data regarding the most common type of cyclical changes. Instead, they appeared to reflect and reproduce a key gender myth: The 'all in the mind' myth that positions all women (but also racialised, or otherwise oppressed populations deemed Other/inferior) as prone to exaggerate/invent/ imagine or manifest experiences. In this case, premenstrual symptoms were positioned by the experts as psychological in essence and origin, rather than predominantly physical in essence and biopsychosocial in origin. This appeared to be a bi-directional and mutually constitutive discursive process (Figure 4.2).

Figure 4.2: The psychologisation of premenstrual changes and reproduction of the 'all in the mind' gender myth

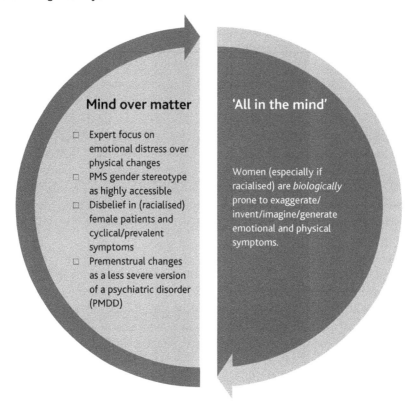

Box 4.1: Mind over matter: why this matters

Science

It turns out that the past 40-plus years of contestation between biomedical and critical PMS research has partly been caused by significantly different definitions of 'PMS'. This situation could easily have been resolved if researchers had collaborated across disciplines, or integrated their research findings, or at least based their descriptions on the available data rather than focusing on psychological changes, only. The prioritisation of emotional distress and minimisation of painful/uncomfortable cyclic changes strongly suggests the (unintentional) influence of the myth of the hysterical/premenstrual female in both critical and biomedical expert accounts of PMS.

Likewise, the biomedical description of PMDD as 'severe PMS' unscientifically positions healthy menstrual physiology as a 'less severe' version of a psychiatric disorder. It is little wonder that both labels have drawn criticism. Given that no specifically 'premenstrual' negative mood change could be identified in a systematic review of prospective studies on mood and the menstrual cycle,[16] there is no scientific basis for implying that cyclic suicidal ideation is a more severe version of mild irritability, or low or anxious mood changes just before, during or after a period.

Clinical practice

Female patients, especially if of a racialised ethnicity, are disproportionately likely to face disbelief in their experiences by clinicians.[17] The myth of the hysterical female/Other, thus, directly contributes to inadequate patient diagnosis and treatment practices, resulting in poorer health outcomes. The psychologisation of cyclical symptoms may also lead biomedical experts to overlook or dismiss descriptions of pain and prevent them from considering physiological causes of discomfort or distress. In turn, this has limited the efficacy and range of treatment options available to patients for decades.

Society

By positioning premenstrual symptoms as largely psychological in origin and type, premenstrual/hysterical/hormonal gender myths are seemingly backed up by biomedical discourses. These myths are known to contribute to many gender inequalities, as described in the first part of this book. While those who have dedicated their careers to helping patients with cyclic symptoms are clearly not doing this on purpose, the creation of non-evidence-based definitions of PMS and PMDD has potentially caused more harm than good.

Personal

I once found a lump in my lower back. I described it to my GP who seemed unimpressed by my concern. Only when he saw how close I was to tears (through sheer frustration) did he bother to 'examine me'. He prodded my back with his finger for less than a couple of seconds then said 'Well, I can't feel anything!'. I felt humiliated. I eventually plucked up the courage to ask to be referred for an ultrasound, to at least rule out the possibility of anything sinister. He very reluctantly did so. In my case, the lump turned out to be a cyst. I still have the cyst and I still remember how I felt during that appointment. I am a six-foot tall, White, middle-class, native English-speaking, tertiary-educated person. If I can be dismissed by a GP about something as obvious as a fatty lump sticking out of my body, I am going to guess that many of you have experienced something similar? It is time to stop the medical dismissal of female (and other marginalised) patients. Exposing and countering the myth of the hysterical/hormonal female or Other is a good place to start.

Snatch-22: premenstrual changes as simultaneously 'normal' and debilitating

This chapter focuses on how the participants described typically mild premenstrual changes versus debilitating cyclical symptoms and the relationship between them. A discursive paradox was identified, which simultaneously implies that 'all women' are necessarily debilitated by the female reproductive body while also minimising individual women's experiences of severe cyclic symptoms. As a result, typically mild premenstrual changes can be positioned as a type of illness, and debilitating cyclic symptoms are positioned as 'normal', creating a problematic *catch-22* situation for female patients, as previously noted by Scambler and Scambler.[1] These contradictory discourses are described here as the 'snatch-22' paradox; partly for ease of reference, but also to emphasise the way in which the female reproductive body is often positioned as *the* marker of, and justification for, women's political inferiority.

Let us start with a look at how and why the participants appeared to both endorse and contest the medicalisation of typical premenstrual changes. We can then move on to similarly contradictory tendencies in relation to the minimisation of severe cyclic symptoms. The third section argues that the way in which typically mild premenstrual changes are positioned *in relation* to debilitating symptoms, and the experts' categorisation of painful physical experiences as something other than Premenstrual Syndrome (PMS) or Premenstrual Dysphoric Disorder (PMDD), unintentionally creates the 'snatch-22' paradox (as well as the belief that premenstrual changes are predominantly psychological in nature).

The medicalisation of typically mild premenstrual changes

As outlined in Chapter 2, the fact that a minority of people experience severe cyclical symptoms can be used to wrongly imply that the menstrual cycle is an inherently debilitating process for most, if not 'all women'. This is what is described within the critical PMS literature as the *medicalisation* or *pathologisation* of the menstrual cycle.[2] This application of debility to an entire gender or sex is also reflected in the PMS stereotype, which positions 'all women' as *pathologically* emotional by virtue of having a female (reproductive) body.

Critical scholars have argued that the creation of female-specific psychiatric disorders (first hysteria now PMDD) reproduces this problematic belief.[3] Especially given that the vast majority of those who menstruate do not experience premenstrual mood changes.[4] They have also challenged the inclusion of typically mild, non-pathological and temporary physical changes in the diagnostic criteria for PMDD (a psychiatric disorder), given that this both medicalises and psychologises the menstrual cycle (highlighted in bold in Table 5.1).

It is not surprising, then, that the three critical experts consistently and explicitly opposed the medicalisation of the menstrual cycle throughout their interviews. For example, in response to a question about their thoughts on the inclusion of non-pathological premenstrual changes in the diagnostic criteria for PMDD.

Yeah, they don't belong there. Ha! [Laugh]. (Geraldine, critical expert [E22])

Table 5.1: The inclusion of typically mild non-pathological changes in the current (DSM V) diagnostic criteria for PMDD

A	In the majority of menstrual cycles, at least five symptoms must be present in the final week before the onset of menses, start to improve within a few days after the onset of menses, and become minimal or absent in the week post menses.
B	One (or more) of the following symptoms must be present: 1. Marked affective lability (e.g., mood swings: feeling suddenly sad or tearful, or increased sensitivity to rejection). 2. Marked irritability or anger or increased interpersonal conflicts. 3. Marked depressed mood, feelings of hopelessness, or self-deprecating thoughts. 4. Marked anxiety, tension, and/or feelings of being keyed up or on edge.
C	One (or more) of the following symptoms must additionally be present, to reach a total of five symptoms when combined with symptoms from Criterion B above. **5. Decreased interest in usual activities (e.g., work, school, friends, hobbies). 6. Subjective difficulty in concentration.** 7. Lethargy, easy fatigability, or marked lack of energy. **8. Marked change in appetite; overeating; or specific food cravings.** 9. Hypersomnia or insomnia. 10. A sense of being overwhelmed or out of control. 11. Physical symptoms such as **breast tenderness or swelling,** joint or muscle pain, **a sensation of 'bloating,' or weight gain.**
Note:	The symptoms in Criteria A–C must have been met for most menstrual cycles that occurred in the preceding year.
D	The symptoms are associated with clinically significant distress or interference with work, school, usual social activities, or relationships with others (e.g., avoidance of social activities; decreased productivity and efficiency at work, school, or home).

Source: APA (2013)

I have thoughts … [about] pathologising menstrual distress as a whole. Yes, I have lots of concerns as to how the diagnosis or how the labelling of PMDD occurs and the classifying of women then, as a result, with a mental health issue. (Zoe, critical expert [E22])

In contrast, the patient and the biomedical expert groups appeared to both endorse *and* contest the medicalisation of non-pathological premenstrual changes, but in different ways.

Contradictory patient discourses

As discussed in the previous chapter, most of the patients included *all* noticeable premenstrual changes in their descriptions of PMS, which associated the healthy menstrual cycle with a biomedical label. This medicalising discourse was apparent throughout the interview data, in the patients' descriptions of their own experiences, as well as in more abstract definitions of PMS in general. For example, when asked how they would describe PMS to someone who had never heard of it before: 'You know, PMS is a collection of symptoms that vary from person to person with a period. You know, it could be anything from mild irritability and weeping all the way to severe cramping, you know, exhaustion? It's just a wide variety of symptoms that kind of vary' (Helen, patient [P13]).

In keeping with this tendency, the patients typically implied that most people who menstruate experience PMS. In fact, in response to a question about the prevalence of PMS, patient estimates ranged from 70 to 100 per cent of women, with a quarter of the group stating that PMS affects 'all women' (of reproductive age). The gendered nature of this discourse illustrates the way in which the patients used the biomedical label of PMS to describe typical non-pathological premenstrual changes of all kinds.

I do believe every woman does have it. (Noor, patient [P14])

Most women, most women, I would think. (Mala, patient [P14])

During the interviews, however, half of the patients also explicitly stated that PMS was 'not an illness', implying that their use of a biomedical label to describe all premenstrual change was perhaps something other than straightforward medicalisation. Indeed, this discourse directly contests the medicalisation of the menstrual cycle, in that it seems to strip the PMS label of its biomedical value.

[I]t's not a disease or an illness. So, like having a period is a natural process and actually I think maybe we need to change the language that we use within health and society … and I don't think it's a disease or an illness. It's just a physical process. (Alice, patient [P15])

Faith: I never thought of it as an illness.
Gemma: Yeah, neither have I, ever! (Faith and Gemma, patients [P29])

This finding is in line with several studies that suggest a significant proportion of those self-identifying as having PMS, even if experiencing debilitating symptoms, do not position it as an illness because the menstrual cycle is considered a healthy experience.[5] In which case, it could be that the patients used the biomedical label simply because 'PMS' is the only term available to them and, therefore, they lacked access to the vocabulary required to differentiate healthy from pathological experiences.

Contradictory expert discourses

Two-thirds of the biomedical experts endorsed the inclusion of non-pathological physical premenstrual changes in the diagnostic criteria for PMDD (a psychiatric disorder), although the strength of their endorsement varied. Four biomedical experts positioned them as less common but relevant and contributing experiences. 'I think there's a place for the physical symptoms, although for most patients, they are not the major issue and not the, the major complaints' (Marta, biomedical expert [E22]). Two biomedical experts qualified their endorsement of the Diagnostic and Statistical Manual of Mental Disorders (DSM) diagnostic criteria by stating that these types of changes only contribute to the PMDD diagnosis if they are moderate to severe.

> So if people are complaining of … breast tenderness and bloating and those are problematic, those would be things that certainly I would consider to be relevant. … But if somebody is just saying those things just happen … and they're not a problem, or happening to a degree that's not that significant, I probably wouldn't count it. (John, biomedical expert [E22])

Finally, as mentioned in the previous chapter, two biomedical experts implied that these typical physical premenstrual changes could even be *caused by* PMDD: 'Many if not all mental diagnoses have physical symptoms. Anxiety is one example of a mental issue that manifests in many physical symptoms' (Barbara, biomedical expert [E22]). One pragmatic explanation for why so many biomedical experts endorsed the inclusion of non-pathological premenstrual changes in the diagnostic criteria for PMDD, however, was that it enables them to support patients who may not otherwise qualify for diagnosis. For instance, without a formal diagnosis, US patients cannot access treatment or healthcare insurance for their cyclical symptoms. Yet, in response to various questions, five of the biomedical experts (plus one critical expert) stated that the current PMDD diagnostic criteria unnecessarily *exclude* some patients who experience severe cyclical mood changes, simply because they do not experience the prerequisite total of five of the 11 listed criteria. Three biomedical experts mentioned this issue when asked to differentiate PMS and PMDD. 'I'm a bit sceptical … for the tendency in DSM to, to demand a certain number of symptoms for this condition [PMDD]. [That] there should be five symptoms. That is, of course, entirely arbitrary … the one [negative mood] symptom, if sufficiently severe, should qualify' (Andrew, biomedical expert [E11]).

It could be that having a minimum number of criteria for a PMDD diagnosis creates an institutional constraint upon clinicians, which is somewhat (but not fully) mitigated by allowing more typical (even if non-pathological) physical premenstrual changes to count towards the diagnosis. By doing so, however, the biomedical experts were unintentionally medicalising such changes and, what is more, positioning them as playing a contributing, if not causal, role in a psychiatric disorder. For example, cyclical suicidal ideation alone does not currently meet the criteria for a diagnosis of PMDD, but if experienced alongside mild premenstrual appetite changes, breast swelling, fatigue, or back pain, it does. This suggests that the current diagnostic criteria are medicalising the menstrual cycle in *two* ways; through the unnecessary inclusion of physical premenstrual changes, and by arbitrarily excluding patients who do not experience such changes alongside severe cyclical mood symptoms.

Crucially, however, five biomedical experts described how it was important to counter the idea that premenstrual changes (of any type) were indicative of a 'disorder'. For instance, in response to a question about the prevalence of PMS, one biomedical expert positioned the problematic attribution of this biomedical label to 'everyone more or less' as a 'lay' discourse, perhaps originating in, and perpetuated by, popular media ('press'): '80 per cent of the female population of fertile age, are not being, have not [got] a disorder. That's something which I have to say. Some lay press it seems, has everyone more or less as having this disorder [PMS], and that's not true' (Thomas, biomedical expert [E5]).

Similarly, when asked what they thought about the inclusion of non-pathological physical changes in the diagnostic criteria for PMDD, five biomedical experts stated that their inclusion was, or could potentially be, a problem. Two explained their position in terms of such changes 'not being part of the PMS/PMDD diagnosis'.

I think it's wrong … those are, are not to be categorised as PMS. (Thomas, biomedical expert [E22])

It's not the physical symptoms that are causing the distress, it's the psychological. So, no [they should not be included in the PMDD criteria]. (Jo, biomedical expert [E22])

Interestingly, the remaining three stated that the inclusion of typically mild premenstrual changes was a concession to, or compromise with, 'the gynaecologists' involved in the formal DSM definition development process for PMDD: '[T]hey do include them, not to annoy the gynaecologists too much, I assume? … I think we should regard item number 11 [typically mild physical changes], in the DSM as a compromise … there's no robust scientific basis for that' (Andrew, biomedical expert [E22]). This type of interdisciplinary tension and subsequent compromise (mainly between psychiatry and gynaecology) was mentioned by several biomedical experts during the interviews. However, all five of the biomedical experts who opposed the inclusion of non-pathological physical premenstrual changes in the diagnostic criteria for PMDD did so on the basis that it was unnecessary, or 'unscientific', rather than explicitly contesting the medicalisation of the menstrual cycle, as such.

Who medicalised what?

Finally, by comparing participant group lists of the 'most common' premenstrual symptoms (in response to question E10/P23), with the robust population data collected by Dennerstein and colleagues,[6] I could discern *which* type of experiences tended to be relatively medicalised (that is, through overemphasis) by the different participant groups (Table 5.2). The three critical experts' responses were combined with those of the biomedical experts because there were too few of them to produce a separate symptom list.

Substantial positive difference in consolidated symptom list position was taken to imply the relative 'medicalisation' of a specific premenstrual change, since this meant they were described at a markedly higher frequency than reported by the general menstruating population (that is, in relation to other common changes). Given that the three symptom lists were of similar length and shared the same 15–18 symptoms, any that were positioned six or more places (that is, over a third of the range) *above* the population data list, were considered indicative of relative medicalisation/overemphasis (shaded entries in Table 5.2). Symptoms mentioned by the participant groups that did not appear on the population study list, and vice versa, are highlighted in bold font.

In keeping with the biomedical and critical experts' tendency to describe PMS as a moderate to severe mood disorder/emotional distress, they mentioned four mood-related symptoms at a substantially higher relative

Table 5.2: The medicalisation of certain premenstrual symptoms listed in order of usage frequency by group and compared to data derived from Dennerstein et al (2011)

	Population data (n=7,226)	All PMS Experts (n=16)	Patients (n=12)
1	Abdominal pain	Irritability/anger	Appetite changes (+9)
2	Irritability	Depression (+9)	Irritability/anger
3	Bloating	Anxiety/tension (+9)	Lack of energy
4	Joint/back/muscle pain	Breast pain	Abdominal pain
5	Breast pain	Bloating	Breast pain
6	Lack of energy	Mood swings	Bloating
7	Headache	Appetite changes	Mood swings
8	Mood swings	Lack of energy	Water retention/weight gain (+6)
9	Anger	Concentration difficulties (+10)	Depression
10	Appetite changes	Sleep disturbance (+8)	Skin changes (+7)
11	Depression	Not in control (+9)	Tearfulness
12	Tension	Hopelessness (suicidal) (+10)	Bowel changes
13	Social withdrawal	Skin changes	**Libido changes**
14	Weight gain (water retention)	**Tearfulness**	Anxiety/ tension
15	Anxiety	Joint/back/muscle pain	Social withdrawal
16	Restlessness	Headache	Joint/back/muscle pain
17	Skin changes	Abdominal pain	Headache
18	Sleep disturbance	Water retention/weight gain	Hopelessness (suicidal)
19	Concentration difficulties	Social withdrawal	**Physical weakness**
20	Not in control	**Dizziness**	**Temperature changes**
21	Swelling of extremities (water retention)	**Increased emotional awareness**	**Bleeding/spotting**
22	Hopelessness (suicidal)		**Cleaning**
23	**Confusion**		

frequency than they occur in the population data. These were 'depression', 'anxiety/tension', feeling 'out of control' and 'suicidal ideation/hopelessness'. The experts also overemphasised 'concentration difficulties' and 'sleep disturbance', two premenstrual changes that were not mentioned *at all* in the patient responses to this question. Interestingly, the premenstrual changes overemphasised by the patients were all typically mild and non-pathological physiological experiences: 'appetite changes', 'water retention/temporary weight gain' and 'skin changes'. The gendered nature of these changes is discussed in the following chapter.

The minimisation of debilitating premenstrual symptoms

The interview participants also appeared to both endorse and contest the *minimisation* of severe cyclic symptoms. Again, the ways in which the different participant groups did so varied.

Contradictory patient discourses

The only minor way in which the patient group endorsed the minimisation of debilitating cyclic symptoms related to half of the group positioning PMS as 'not an illness'. While this discourse primarily contests the medicalisation of the healthy menstrual cycle, it also contributes to the minimisation of severe symptoms in that it could be implied that, if cyclic, they are not a serious or 'real' health issue. While this was clearly not the intention of the patients, their apparent lack of access to alternative terms with which to differentiate typical changes from debilitating symptoms (usually indicative of underlying conditions) created a contradiction, which likely contributes to the snatch-22 paradox. In fact, one of the patients explicitly demonstrated this discursive dilemma.

> Yeah, I think if someone's experiencing very extreme symptoms as a result of their period, then there's definitely some, you know, it's a condition. I don't know what the term would be? Um, and then maybe it wouldn't be called an illness, but I'd want it to be recognised properly. Um, I wouldn't want to say it's not an illness just because I don't suffer it in the same way [laugh]. (Kathleen, patient [P30])

A far more common patient concern was that other people may disbelieve, or otherwise dismiss or minimise, premenstrual experiences. It was, therefore, not surprising that the patient group also contested the minimisation of debilitating cyclic symptoms. All but two of the group explicitly positioned such minimisation as a problem because it can prevent individuals from accessing adequate support or treatment.

> I think they [doctors] dismiss it as just something got to do with hormones? ... Some people go through really, really bad stages of PMS where ... they can't control themselves at all ... and there's not really an explanation or help for it. (Mala, patient [P17])

> Sometimes I feel like I'm teaching them [doctors] and then they call me an 'expert patient' or whatever they call it. I think it's just seen too much as a norm. (Aisha, patient [P18])

This concern did not appear to be unfounded. For example, four out of five of the patients who had consulted doctors about debilitating cyclic symptoms described how their experiences were (initially) minimised and, thus, deemed not to require examination, diagnosis or treatment. It is worth mentioning that all four were eventually diagnosed with underlying health conditions.

> I was told 'this is all in your head' [severe abdominal pain and negative mood changes] … I was never given like a consistent straight thing outside of 'Go home, take a Midol, go shopping, you'll feel better'. (Helen, patient, eventually diagnosed with PMDD and fibroids [P17])

> Yeah. I have [consulted doctors] but they don't suggest anything for it [cyclical suicidal ideation]. I've never got anything for it. (Aisha, patient, eventually diagnosed with Borderline Personality Disorder [P17])

Two of the patients were dismissed despite experiencing vomiting and fainting due to extreme pelvic pain. These symptoms are usually (and were in both cases) indicative of underlying gynaecological conditions such as endometriosis, iron-deficiency anaemia and/or fibroids.

> I had vomited and had diarrhoea all over the place and I passed out in the middle of a shopping mall … and my dad and sister arrived to find me in this heap … so they rushed me to see a GP … and he just said … 'Yeah, you're fine now, everything's fine, go home and rest'. (Alice, patient, eventually diagnosed with endometriosis [P17])

> The first time I went to the hospital [with severe uterine pain, vomiting and having fainted], um, they said it was food poisoning [laugh] without even examining me, they were just like 'Oh yeah, it's food poisoning. Have a paracetamol and go home'. … Next time, again, without examining me, he told me it was a UTI [urinary tract infection]. (Faith, patient, eventually diagnosed with fibroids, ovarian cysts and iron-deficiency anaemia [P17])

Contradictory expert discourses

For the biomedical experts, specific references to, or examples of, the *minimisation* of debilitating cyclic symptoms were far less common. Nearly half of the group, however, did mention the 'clinical dismissal' of premenstrual symptoms and positioned this as a key issue for patients.

> I started to see patients and one of the things that was really striking is that they were in a great deal of distress. They had a lot of trouble finding people who believed them and even more trouble finding people that had some (pause) reasonable, er, you know, could articulate some reasonable treatment options for them. (Laura, biomedical expert [E1])

> There are lots of reasons why you might not be asked [about a cyclical symptom pattern], sort of practical reasons, but also ignorance … because there is a history of not believing female patients about these sorts of experiences. (Jo, biomedical expert [E17])

Importantly, a biomedical-specific discourse was identified in the interview data that may contribute to the minimisation of (some) debilitating premenstrual symptoms (as well as their psychologisation). Nearly half of the biomedical expert group seemed to position physical premenstrual symptoms as *inherently* less debilitating, or distressing, than negative mood ones. 'Many women do have somatic symptoms, but don't regard them as very problematic' (Andrew, biomedical expert [E10]). Crucially, these biomedical experts were all referencing the type of patients *who come to see them* regarding severe PMS or PMDD, rather than the population data regarding problematic premenstrual changes in the general population. Indeed, a couple of them used disclaimers ('certainly the people … I see' and 'I rarely see …') that made the specific clinical context of this perspective explicit.

> In reality (pause) certainly the people who come to this [psychiatric] clinic and I see are here because of the psychological, far more than the physical [symptoms]. (John, biomedical expert [E9])

> I'm just saying, I rarely see anybody who is functionally impaired by just physical symptoms. (Laura, biomedical expert [E20])

Positioning painful physical symptoms as inherently 'less debilitating' than those relating to mood illustrates the disconnect between (epidemiologically consistent) patient and (psychologised) expert definitions of PMS. For example, four out of the five patients who had consulted a doctor about their premenstrual symptoms (which to them constituted PMS), described doing so in relation to severe physical changes only, or as well as, negative mood changes (highlighted in Table 5.3). Contrary to biomedical expert

Table 5.3: Have you ever consulted a doctor about your premenstrual symptoms? Patient data disclosed during interviews

Patient	Premenstrual symptom(s)	Severity described	Consulted doctor?	Related/eventual diagnosis
Aisha	Low and irritable mood, suicidal ideation	Severe	Yes	Borderline Personality Disorder
Alice	Abdominal pain	Severe	Yes	Endometriosis
Emma	Low/irritable mood and abdominal pain	Severe	Yes	PMDD and IBS
Faith	Abdominal pain	Severe	Yes	Fibroids and iron-deficiency anaemia
Helen	Low/irritable mood and abdominal pain	Severe	Yes	PMDD and fibroids
Beth	Exacerbation of anxiety	Moderate-severe	No	Generalised anxiety disorder
Dani	Fatigue	Moderate	No	n/a
Gemma	Digestive issues and low self-esteem	Mild–moderate	No	n/a
Kathleen	Abdominal pain and low mood	Mild–moderate	No	Fibroids, iron-deficiency anaemia
Mala	Appetite changes	Mild–moderate	No	n/a
Noor	Irritable mood and appetite changes	Mild–moderate	No	Iron-deficiency anaemia
Ria	Social withdrawal, low libido and appetite changes	Mild–moderate	No	n/a

discourses, therefore, it appears to have been the *severity* rather than *type* of premenstrual symptom that motivated help–seeking behaviour.

The critical experts did not tend to directly reference or describe examples of the minimisation of severe cyclic symptoms, but one of them positioned the clinical dismissal of patients as problematic. At times, all three of the critical experts appeared to downplay the potential severity of cyclic symptoms, although this seemed to be due to their more accurate categorisation of such symptoms as something 'other' than PMS, rather than straightforward minimisation. For example, in response to a question about how best to 'manage PMS', Geraldine implied that patient self-care (lines 1 and 2) and improved understanding of premenstrual change (lines 3 and 4) would be enough to alleviate premenstrual symptoms without the need for, in her opinion, 'invalid' medical intervention (line 2) (Excerpt 5.1). This could be interpreted as a form of minimisation.

Excerpt 5.1

1 [Pause] let's see (.) probably with self-care (.) extra rest (.) stress
2 management (.) um (.) things like that (.) I mean, there isn't really any valid medical
3 treatment (.) so I would say self-care and probably you know (.) if women could be
4 taught some cognitive therapy or you know (.) some feminist analysis so they could
5 <u>rethink</u> what the symptoms mean (.) I think they would be able to manage them and
6 feel better.
   (Geraldine, critical expert [E7])

In response to a later question, however, Geraldine clarified her position as referring only to those *without* any underlying conditions or distress. For her (as well as the other two critical experts), severe negative mood changes such as suicidal ideation were typically positioned as necessarily indicative of something other than typical premenstrual change or PMS (a perspective in line with the available data).

[T]hat's not to say that no women suffer … it's possible that those women might have experience of trauma early in life that could relate to this. It's possible that they have a form of depression that waxes and wanes and is affected by biochemical changes associated with the menstrual cycle. So, they may feel suicidal at certain times of the month, but maybe generally depressed overall … and so treatment really has to be related to individual patients. (Geraldine, critical expert [E17])

Who minimised what?

Finally, as before, by comparing the expert and patient group lists of the 'most common premenstrual symptoms' with population data,[7] I could discern which symptoms were relatively minimised (that is, through underemphasis) by the participant groups (shaded entries in Table 5.4). Again, the three critical experts' responses were combined with those of the clinicians. Any symptoms ranked six or more places *below* the epidemiological data list (over a third of the range), were considered indicative of 'relative minimisation'.

Other than breast pain and bloating, pain-related experiences were more likely to be underemphasised than other types of premenstrual change. Indeed, 'headache' (nine positions lower) and 'joint/back/muscle pain' (11 positions lower) were similarly minimised by both the patient and expert groups. This may be because both symptoms are relatively easily managed with over-the-counter painkillers.

Only 'abdominal pain' stands out as a major difference between the population and patient lists, and that of the experts (16 positions lower) (Table 5.4). The tendency of the experts to minimise abdominal/uterine

Table 5.4: The minimisation of certain premenstrual symptoms listed in order of usage frequency by group and compared to data derived from Dennerstein et al (2011)

	Population data (n=7,226)	All experts (n=16)	Patients (n=12)
1	Abdominal pain	Irritability/anger	Appetite changes
2	Irritability	Depression	Irritability/anger
3	Bloating	Anxiety/tension	Lack of energy
4	Joint/back/muscle pain	Breast pain	Abdominal pain
5	Breast pain	Bloating	Breast pain
6	Lack of energy	Mood swings	Bloating
7	Headache	Appetite changes	Mood swings
8	Mood swings	Lack of energy	Water retention/weight gain
9	Anger	Concentration difficulties	Depression
10	Appetite changes	Sleep disturbance	Skin changes
11	Depression	Not in control	Tearfulness
12	Tension	Hopelessness (suicidal)	Bowel changes
13	Social withdrawal	Skin changes	**Libido changes**
14	Weight gain (water retention)	**Tearfulness**	Anxiety/tension
15	Anxiety	Joint/back/muscle pain (-11)	Social withdrawal
16	Restlessness	Headache (-9)	Joint/back/muscle pain (-11)
17	Skin changes	Abdominal pain (-16)	Headache (-9)
18	Sleep disturbance	Water retention/weight gain	Hopelessness (suicidal)
19	Concentration difficulties	Social withdrawal	**Physical weakness**
20	Not in control	**Dizziness**	**Temperature changes**
21	Swelling of extremities (water retention)	**Increased emotional awareness**	**Bleeding/spotting**
22	Hopelessness (suicidal)		**Cleaning**
23	**Confusion**		

pain is easy to explain. When asked if they considered period pain (the lay term for cyclical abdominal/uterine pain) to be a premenstrual symptom, around two-thirds of the experts (biomedical and critical experts alike) stated that they did not because it occurs during menstruation and so belongs to a separate diagnostic category. Seven of the experts labelled this '*dysmenorrhea*'. By categorising abdominal pain as something other than PMS, the experts were less likely to include it as part of the PMS diagnosis.

No, I wouldn't because I'm a gynaecologist. I would say that's dysmenorrhea or potentially endometriosis. (Marta, biomedical expert [E12])

No. I see it as a menstrual symptom. Um, if you're talking about period pain, then there are changes pre period, which are menstrual symptoms, but no, I don't consider period pain a PMS, to be a PMS symptom, no. (Zoe, critical expert [E12])

In contrast, all but two of the patients *did* count period pain as a PMS symptom, which explains why 'abdominal pain' appeared high up in their symptom list, in line with the population data (Table 5.3). The patients (and the remaining third of the expert group) also tended to justify their position in relation to the timing of period pain. In this case, because it often occurs in the days *before* menstruation, as supported by prospective epidemiological studies of dysmenorrhea.[8]

Debbie: Yes, if they're [period cramps] premenstrual [laugh]
Interviewer: So, it's just the timing?
Debbie: Yeah. (Debbie, biomedical expert [E12])

Oh, yeah, yeah. I think for a lot of women, it can be that the pain they get associated with the period starts before the menstrual flow starts. Yeah. (Beth, patient [P24])

Constructing the 'snatch-22' paradox

As discussed earlier, the participants used discourses that both contested *and* endorsed the medicalisation *and* minimisation of certain premenstrual experiences. This section describes a couple of key discursive mechanisms that appear to enable such contradictory discourses to simultaneously exist. Namely, the use of 'normal curve' analogies to describe the relationship between non-pathological changes and severe cyclic symptoms, and the biomedical categorisation of severe physical symptoms as something other than PMS or PMDD. It is argued that these two mechanisms help to create and perpetuate the snatch-22 paradox, whereby typical premenstrual changes are sometimes positioned as pathological, while debilitating cyclic symptoms (indicative of an underlying condition) are sometimes positioned as 'normal'.

The use of normal curve analogies

Most of the participants (11 out of the 13 biomedical experts, two out of the three critical experts, and nine out of the 12 patients) employed a 'normal curve' analogy when describing the way in which premenstrual experiences vary considerably between individuals. For instance, four of the biomedical experts explicitly described a normal 'bell curve' or 'spectrum' of experience when differentiating PMS from PMDD.

> I think that by the time somebody gets to a level of severity, you know, sort of this like bell curve, right? Of you've got PMS somewhere down here and then it turns into PMDD. (Debbie, biomedical expert [E11])

> To me, PMDD is at the most severe end of the spectrum of premenstrual symptoms. (Fran, biomedical expert [E11])

Similarly, Susan, a critical expert, positioned 'significant' distress (line 3) as 'part of' (line 2) 'normal' premenstrual change (line 2), when asked how she would describe PMS to someone who had not heard of it before.

> What I would say is 'Well, women expect change over the menstrual cycle, that's quite normal' ... a smaller proportion of women who experience distress as part of that change and distress that might have a significant impact on their lives and that that is often referred to as PMS. (Susan, critical expert [E2])

The patients typically implied a normal curve or spectrum of experience discourse by positioning debilitating changes as a more 'extreme' or 'intense' version of normal premenstrual changes or PMS. For instance, when asked to differentiate PMDD from PMS.

> I think that it [PMDD] is a much more extreme version where like the person suffering from it can actually feel suicidal and (pause) incredibly unstable and unhappy at certain times? (Dani, patient [P20])

> PMDD, I don't know, but I think that one is more of the intense one? (Noor, patient [P20])

Although, one patient did explicitly employ a 'normal curve' analogy when asked how they would describe PMS to someone who had not heard of it: 'But like looking at the normal curve and distribution, a lot of PMS quote unquote "symptoms" are just things [laugh] that happen to us during that time, which are like beautiful and magical' (Ria, patient [P13]). Crucially, the empirical data do not imply a 'normal curve' from none or very mild premenstrual changes all the way to cyclic suicidal thinking and/or excruciating period pain. Indeed, just within this small study, all five of the patients who consulted doctors about their severe premenstrual symptoms were eventually diagnosed with underlying health conditions.

Plus, as previously discussed, cyclic suicidal ideation or severe mood swings are most likely the exacerbation of underlying distress. Similarly, regularly severe period pain that does not respond to lifestyle changes, hormonal suppression or anti-inflammatory medications is automatically classified as *secondary* dysmenorrhea.[9] By definition, this 'secondary' diagnosis confirms that it is most likely caused by an underlying condition, such as fibroids, endometriosis, adenomyosis, or pelvic inflammatory disease, and so not merely a more severe version of period pain (uterine cramps).[10] There is, therefore, no scientific rationale for positioning regularly severe cyclic symptoms of *any* type at the far end of a 'normal range' of premenstrual changes.

The problem is that by positioning severe cyclic symptoms such as suicidal behaviour, or excruciating abdominal pain, at the far end of a normally distributed curve, or spectrum, of typical experiences, all premenstrual changes become imbued with (potential) pathology (that is, the medicalisation of the menstrual cycle). At the same time, severe cyclical symptoms can be positioned as simply 'more severe' versions of (non-pathological) premenstrual changes, which effectively obscures the underlying conditions being triggered or exacerbated (that is, the minimisation of debilitating cyclic symptoms). In this way, these analogies help construct and perpetuate the snatch-22 paradox.

For instance, when asked how she would describe PMS to someone who had not heard of it before, one biomedical expert demonstrated how the normal curve analogy can only superficially differentiate mild changes from debilitating cyclic symptoms since it implies that they are both part of the same (inherently pathological) physiological experience (Excerpt 5.2).

Excerpt 5.2

1 PMS is (.) is (.) is very mild (pause) symptoms in the two weeks
2 before menses [...] it's a (.) it's a (.) it's a nuisance only (.) nothing more than
3 mild nuisance [...] but I guess it's hard for me to answer that question without
4 talking about PMDD because I think of them as a sort of continuum? (.) but I
5 really conceptualise anything that is impairing or significantly distressing at all
6 (.) as a PMDD symptom (.) whereas PMS (.) I would say (.) is not disordered
7 (.) it's just sort of (.) little mild changes that are not of any consequence (.)
8 and don't really bother you.
   (Debbie, biomedical expert [E2])

Debbie's use of the analogy ('continuum', line 4) appeared to make it difficult for her to describe PMS (which to her refers to typically mild changes, only), without referencing PMDD (line 4). This suggests that the normal curve analogy directly limits a speaker's ability to accurately differentiate non-pathological premenstrual changes from debilitating symptoms, even though the latter are indicative of underlying health conditions.

Another biomedical expert, Sarah, illustrated the other side of the snatch-22 paradox (the minimisation/normalisation of severe cyclic symptoms) in response to a question about how best to manage PMS (Excerpt 5.3).

Excerpt 5.3

1 [O]f course there are more severe syndromes [...] we had a woman in our
2 ward who um (.) I was asked to see because she was self-immolating (.) she was
3 you know (.) she was psychotic and um (.) tried to set fire to herself at menses (.) and
4 it was (.) the problem was (.) she had um (.) four young children (.) she was (.) you
5 know (.) a baby six months old or something (.) and her sister had successfully set
6 fire to herself and died the year before in our ward [...] and we (.) I suppressed her
7 cycle using very potent you know (.) medications (.) we didn't have GNRH analogues
8 then but something (.) something similar (.) Danazole (.) and the whole thing
9 stopped! and before that [softly laughing, shaking head] I'm telling you (.) it was still
10 happening despite giving her the oral contraceptive pill to suppress the cycle (.) it
11 wasn't suppressing the cycle and she was (.) and she was still doing it.
   (Sarah, biomedical expert [E7])

In response to a question about PMS, Sarah described treating a 'psychotic' patient (line 3) who repeatedly attempted suicide during her period ('at menses', line 3). She positioned the patient's experiences as a 'more severe syndrome' (line 1) implying that this behaviour is a more extreme version of PMS/normal premenstrual changes (normal curve analogy), rather than the premenstrual exacerbation (PME) of psychosis/severe emotional distress. Sarah effectively positions the patient's attempts at self-immolation as mainly due to her healthy reproductive biology ('I suppressed her cycle ... and the whole thing stopped!', lines 6–8; and 'it wasn't suppressing the cycle ... and she was still doing it', lines 10–11), undermining the role of several contributing psychosocial factors ('four young children ...' and 'her sister had successfully set fire to herself ...', lines 4–6) and the fact that she was presumably ill enough during the rest of her menstrual cycle to warrant ongoing hospitalisation within a psychiatric 'ward' (lines 2 and 6). Again, it seems as though the normal curve analogy actively limited Sarah's ability to discursively differentiate the PME of psychosis from PMS/non-pathological premenstrual changes.

Crucially, other types of exacerbated conditions, such as menstrual migraine or catamenial epilepsy, were not typically positioned as 'more severe' versions of typical premenstrual changes. For example, when asked if exacerbated conditions counted as premenstrual symptoms, 11 of the 13 biomedical experts and two of the three critical experts described these experiences as *fundamentally different* to PMS/PMDD. (As mentioned in the previous chapter, all but two of the patients were demonstrably unaware of the concept of PME when asked the same question.)

> Um, no, but I think it's, it's fair to say that a number of disorders are, can be worsened by the menstrual cycle and you need to be aware of that. I don't think they are specific Premenstrual Syndromes, though. (Sarah, biomedical expert [E14])

> Um, generally, no. … These things may be exacerbated but I would not view them as premenstrual symptoms. (Zoe, critical expert [E14])

Different diagnoses for severe physical premenstrual symptoms

A second discursive mechanism also contributes to the catch-22 paradox: the existence of alternative biomedical diagnoses for debilitating physical premenstrual symptoms, which effectively removes them from the PMS label, especially if they are the main or sole complaint. Just as severe period pain is given the label 'dysmenorrhea', most cyclical physical symptoms (if severe) can be diagnosed as something other than PMS. For instance, severe premenstrual bloating, constipation and/or diarrhoea can be labelled (premenstrually exacerbated) 'irritable bowel syndrome' (IBS), severe headache can be labelled '(menstrual) migraine' and severe breast pain can be labelled 'mastalgia' (Table 5.5).

In addition, severe physical symptoms are also relatively easily managed by the patient alone, or with the support of their GP, and so are less likely to involve a specialist PMS clinician (either a psychiatrist or gynaecologist). In fact, most physical symptoms respond well to first-line treatments, such as lifestyle interventions (nutritional supplements, anti-inflammatory diet and stress reduction), or contraceptive, diuretic or anti-inflammatory medications.[11] Even if the problem persists (indicating an underlying condition), aside from uterine pain and breast pain, debilitating physical premenstrual symptoms are also more likely to be referred to 'non-PMS' clinical specialisms, such as neurology or gastroenterology (Table 5.5). In this way, most severe physical premenstrual symptoms are effectively removed from the oversight of gynaecology and psychiatry, and PMS research. This also helps to explain why the biomedical PMS experts discursively positioned physical symptoms as 'less common' and inherently 'less debilitating' than mood changes.

Chapter summary

The expert and patient descriptions of PMS proved extremely useful in explaining how and why certain premenstrual experiences were prioritised over others (and by whom). A novel finding of this study was

Table 5.5: The biomedical labelling of, and clinical specialism responsible for, the top 20 most common premenstrual changes

#	Premenstrual symptom	Alternative diagnostic label if main complaint and debilitating	Clinical specialism typically responsible
5	Breast pain	Mastalgia/mastodynia	GP
6	Lack of energy	Anaemia/insomnia	GP
9	Appetite changes	Eating disorder	GP
14	Restlessness	Restless leg syndrome/anaemia	GP
18	Swelling of extremities	Oedema	GP
3	Bloating (digestive pain)	IBS/food intolerance digestive issue	GP/Gastroenterology
4	Joint/back/ muscle pain	Musculoskeletal injury/ rheumatism	GP/Rheumatology/ Physiotherapy
7	Headache	Headache/migraine/neurological issue	GP/Neurology
13	Weight gain	Poor nutrition/lack of exercise	GP/Dietician
15	Skin changes	Acne/eczema/psoriasis	GP/Dermatology
16	Sleep disturbance	Insomnia/hypersomnia	GP/Sleep specialist
17	Concentration difficulties	Anaemia/insomnia/neurological issue	GP/Neurology
20	Confusion	Anaemia/insomnia/neurological issue	GP/Neurology
1	Abdominal (uterine) pain	Dysmenorrhea/endometriosis/pelvic inflammatory disease/fibroids	GP/Gynaecology
2	Irritability/anger	PMS/PMDD or depression/anxiety	GP/Gynaecology/Psychiatry
8	Mood swings/ not in control	PMS/PMDD or depression/anxiety	GP/Gynaecology/Psychiatry
10	Depression	PMS/PMDD or depression	GP/Gynaecology/Psychiatry
11	Tension/anxiety	PMS/PMDD or anxiety	GP/Gynaecology/Psychiatry
12	Social withdrawal	PMS/PMDD or depression/anxiety	GP/Gynaecology/Psychiatry
19	Hopelessness (suicidal)	PMS/PMDD or depression	GP/Gynaecology/Psychiatry

that contrary to much of the PMS literature, there was no straightforward binary opposition between 'biomedical' and 'feminist academic' discourses regarding the medicalisation of the menstrual cycle. Over a third of the biomedical experts also mentioned concerns about labelling typically mild and/or non-pathological premenstrual changes as PMS or PMDD, albeit due to this being 'unscientific' rather than medicalising, as such. Medicalising discourses were, however, still endorsed by most of the biomedical experts, for example, the positioning of several typically mild and non-pathological premenstrual changes as constitutive symptoms of PMDD (a psychiatric disorder), contrary to the available evidence base.

In keeping with their typical descriptions of PMS, the biomedical experts relatively medicalised premenstrual mood changes and minimised pain-related ones. Several of the biomedical experts also positioned physical cyclic symptoms as inherently 'less debilitating', a discourse not borne out by patient accounts in this study or the population data. This perspective appeared to be informed by the type of patients PMS-specialist clinicians consult, the existence of alternative diagnoses and treatment pathways for physical complaints, and the fact that they are more easily managed at the primary care level.

The critical experts explicitly and consistently contested the medicalisation of the menstrual cycle and the minimisation of debilitating symptoms, on the basis that they reinforced problematic and discriminatory gender beliefs and practices. However, they did still (unintentionally) relatively medicalise mood changes and minimise premenstrual pain. The group also occasionally appeared to downplay the potential severity of cyclic symptoms, but this was due to their positioning of them as necessarily indicative of 'other' underlying conditions, emotional distress or trauma, in line with the available population data.

The patients used the biomedical label 'PMS' to describe all noticeable premenstrual changes (regardless of severity) and overestimated its population prevalence, which were both unintentionally 'medicalising' discourses. However, half of the patients also explicitly stated that PMS was 'not an illness', thus explicitly contesting medicalisation (and perhaps even unintentionally minimising debilitating cyclic symptoms) by removing the label's biomedical value. This suggests that the group's reliance on the term PMS is perhaps indicative of a lack of access to alternative vocabulary with which to describe non-pathological premenstrual changes, or the premenstrual exacerbation of underlying conditions (PME). The patients relatively medicalised three highly gendered physical changes (temporary appetite, weight and skin changes) in comparison to the population data.

In short, participant discourses were not based on the available data regarding the most common premenstrual symptoms or the non-linear relationship between typical premenstrual changes and regularly severe cyclic symptoms (indicative of underlying health conditions). Instead, a couple of discursive devices were identified, which appeared to help construct a 'snatch-22' paradox, whereby non-pathological premenstrual changes can be medicalised, while debilitating cyclic symptoms (indicative of underlying conditions) can be minimised/normalised. The main device being the use of 'normal curve' analogies to inaccurately describe the relationship between typical changes and severe cyclic symptoms. The second device being alternative biomedical labels for severe physical symptoms, which effectively removes them from the PMS label and associated clinical specialisms (Figure 5.1).

Figure 5.1: Premenstrual changes as simultaneously 'normal' and debilitating

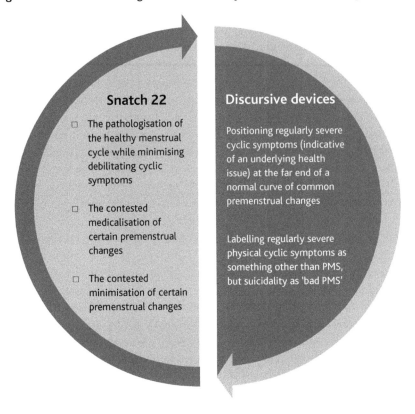

Snatch 22

☐ The pathologisation of the healthy menstrual cycle while minimising debilitating cyclic symptoms

☐ The contested medicalisation of certain premenstrual changes

☐ The contested minimisation of certain premenstrual changes

Discursive devices

Positioning regularly severe cyclic symptoms (indicative of an underlying health issue) at the far end of a normal curve of common premenstrual changes

Labelling regularly severe physical cyclic symptoms as something other than PMS, but suicidality as 'bad PMS'

Box 5.1: Snatch-22: why this matters

Science

The inaccurate application of a scientific term such as 'normal curve' to describe the relationship between healthy (albeit disruptive and uncomfortable) physiological processes and regularly severe cyclic symptoms has had far-reaching negative consequences. It also seems to have restricted scientific research into healthy menstrual physiology and the likely (inflammatory) causes of typical premenstrual changes, as well as the cyclic exacerbation of many underlying conditions.

Clinical practice

The 'normal curve' analogy has no doubt contributed to inadequate diagnostic and treatment practices regarding a wide range of female-prevalent health conditions. For instance, the typical (several years) delay in diagnosis (often due to the medical dismissal of female patients/symptoms) of endometriosis, Polycystic Ovary Syndrome, fibromyalgia, ME or PMDD. The arbitrary and problematic biomedical prioritisation of premenstrual emotional distress over (far more common) experiences of pain, also serves to psychologise female patients, their symptoms and these health conditions.

Society

The creation of a female-specific (and reproductive) psychiatric disorder, without an adequate evidence base, is highly reminiscent of earlier medical/societal discourses around female hysteria. By positioning PMDD as something 'other' than an underlying condition triggered or worsened by the menstrual cycle (as suggested by the available data), premenstrual changes of all types are also effectively psychologised and pathologised. This has the dual effect of minimising female pain and positioning 'all women' as inherently (pathologically) emotional due to the menstrual cycle. Given that menstrual migraine, cyclic asthma and catamenial epilepsy are not positioned as being on the far end of a 'normal curve' of premenstrual changes, it appears as though severe emotional distress (including suicidal ideation) has been categorised differently, simply because it fits an existing gender myth.

Personal

As the 'snatch-22' paradox identifies, we currently cannot win when it comes to our menstrual health (or illness). The use of normal curve analogies allows the minimisation and normalisation of regularly severe and debilitating cyclic symptoms (typically indicative of an underlying health issue), while also positioning 'all women' as inherently (mentally and physically) debilitated by the healthy functioning of the menstrual cycle. Nobody positions the symptoms of coeliac disease as 'severe digestion' or asthma as 'severe respiration' and yet, too many of us think of endometriosis or PMDD as 'bad periods' or 'severe PMS'. This must stop.

6

The curse: femininity as debility

This chapter examines the ways in which gender myths appeared to inform participant descriptions of the cause(s), prevalence and management of Premenstrual Syndrome (PMS), as well as the prioritisation of certain premenstrual changes over others. The first part focuses on how and why the participants positioned the female sex hormones as the main *cause* of debilitating cyclical symptoms, contrary to the available scientific data. Then I will discuss the way in which certain types of premenstrual change, and biomedical treatment options, were prioritised due to pervasive gender norms. The last section describes how and why the participants tended to exaggerate the prevalence and number of debilitating premenstrual symptoms in the general menstruating population, which (unintentionally) implies that the female (reproductive) body is inherently debilitating.

Blaming the female sex (hormones)

Starting with the biomedical experts, when asked to explain why premenstrual symptoms occur, two-thirds of the group provided biological explanations only (without any reference to external psychosocial factors). A third of the biomedical expert group specifically attributed *causality* to the female sex hormones, especially progesterone and/or its metabolites.[1]

Laura:	I think it's a hormonal withdrawal effect that, er, leads to some changes in neurotransmitter signal, signalling.
Interviewer:	Any specific hormone or all of the ones involved in the menstrual cycle?
Laura:	Er, I don't think we know. Um, it's more likely, I think, to be progesterone and progesterone metabolites? (Laura, biomedical expert [E6])

It is either progesterone occurring, sorry, stimulating somewhere in the brain because of the close relationship with progesterone production following ovulation. Um, or it may be a metabolic by product/ breakdown product of progesterone such as allopregnanolone and pregnanolone. (Chris, biomedical expert [E6])

As discussed in the first part of this book, the attribution of direct causation to either of the female sex hormones (oestrogen and progestogen or their metabolites) in PMS/Premenstrual Dysphoric Disorder (PMDD) is not supported by the available data, despite numerous attempts to identify such a relationship over the past 90 years. What is more, since the 1980s, it has been consistently established that the (male and female) sex hormone levels of those with or without PMS/PMDD symptoms do not differ.[2] This suggests that there is no 'hormonal' abnormality in those experiencing cyclical symptoms, therefore, they are unlikely to play a main or sole causal role.

Two-thirds of the biomedical experts thus employed a slightly amended version of the hormonal discourse. They still positioned the female sex hormones as the main causal factor in symptoms, but as mediated by an (ill-defined) abnormal genetic and/or neurological 'sensitivity' in PMS/PMDD patients. In this way, the positioning of the female sex hormones as potentially, if not inherently, pathological remained, despite acknowledging that there must be something fundamentally *different* about those who experienced debilitating cyclic symptoms.

> So it seems to be to do with sensitivity to either, you know, hormones or neurotransmitters. ... It's not like there's any measurable difference between women who are affected or unaffected, but it is to do with that individual's response. (Jo, biomedical expert [E6])

> I think some people may be more sensitive to the progestogen increase that occurs at the time of ovulation premenstrually. I think for some people it might be the drop in oestrogen that occurs. I think for other people it's potentially something else, er, indirectly related to one or other of those things. (John, biomedical expert [E6])

Additionally, when asked to compare male and female experiences of (non-sex-specific) symptoms associated with PMS, two-thirds of the biomedical experts implied that exactly the same symptoms (whether cyclical or not) have *fundamentally* different causal mechanisms, depending upon an individual's sex. Tellingly, two-thirds of the biomedical experts *only* described negative mood symptoms in their responses to this question.

Excerpt 6.1

1 [M]en do have hormones circulating and you know (.) testosterone [...] but I
2 would say the big difference is that their levels are more stable [...] but the
3 intrinsic difference between men and women as well (.) that they er (.) I'm

4 very much generalising now (.) but they often react to things in different ways
5 (.) perhaps emotionally [...] like Venus and Mars! [Laugh].
(Anne, biomedical expert [E16])

The fact that both female sex hormone levels and moods can 'fluctuate' appeared to be interpreted as suggestive of a causal association between them ('men ... are more stable' in lines 1 and 2) (Excerpt 6.1). Anne went on to imply another 'intrinsic' (line 2) sex difference in the way in which individuals 'react to things' (line 4), by referencing a (scientifically debunked[3]) pop-psychology book that positions cisgender men and women as having categorically different (that is, biologically determined) psychological profiles ('like Venus and Mars', line 5) (Excerpt 6.1). Her use of a disclaimer ('I'm very much generalising now' in lines 3 and 4) suggested some awareness that this idea is stereotypical rather than scientific, but she continued to position it as a *causal* factor in these symptoms.

In fact, most of the biomedical experts described sex differences in the *causes* of low mood, using the circular argument that cisgender men do not have the same 'fluctuations' in female sex hormones. This overlooks the fact that around half of the female population is not of reproductive age[4] and so does not experience 'fluctuating levels' of these sex hormones, and of those who do, over 90 per cent do not typically experience problematic negative mood symptoms.[5] 'I would assume that in women it is due to the interaction between their neurotransmitters and hormonal fluctuations and in men, uh, they don't have hormonal fluctuations in the same way ... I think they're different because in women the symptoms are because of a vulnerability to hormonal fluctuations' (Fran, biomedical expert [E16]).

Tellingly, one biomedical expert appeared to suggest that his own study's finding that the male partners of PMS patients experienced *concurrent* negative mood changes, revealed some sort of 'psychological' response to their partner's 'biological' experiences. I would argue that this finding is far more likely to reflect shared distressing experiences, than some sort of mysterious sympathetic psychosomatic phenomenon: 'We did ... a study on [male] partners and ... they did daily ratings and they showed a similar pattern in their mood as their [female] partners. ... Well, in that case, in those men, I think it is psychological, it's not biological' (Thomas, biomedical expert [E16]).

The (hysterical/hormonal female) gender myth that attributes cis women's emotions to their reproductive body, thus, appeared to influence the biomedical experts' descriptions of the causes of cyclical symptoms when forced to compare them with male experiences of exactly the same symptoms. Given that PMS and PMDD are formally defined as *biopsychosocial* conditions, the overriding dominance of the biological 'hormonal' causal discourse in the biomedical expert descriptions seemed disproportionate, and again based more on gender myths than the available data.

The uptake of biomedical discourses by others

In contrast, all three of the critical experts mentioned biological, psychological and social factors as contributing factors in cyclic symptoms. In fact, they tended to highlight the role of external psychosocial factors as the *main* cause of emotional distress, positioning the menstrual cycle as more of an 'exacerbating' or 'contributing' factor. 'So there's definitely something physiological that's occurring, but it's that interaction with what's actually happening in the woman's experience, in the woman's life and emotionally that makes the difference, I think' (Zoe, critical expert [E6]).

Interestingly, however, when describing the 'biological' element, the critical experts also typically referred to (the female sex) 'hormones'. Again, this could have been due to the group's tendency to quote biomedical discourses when discussing embodied changes.

> I would take what some might call a biopsychosocial approach … hormonal changes can lead to, or can be associated with, changes in how a woman experiences her body … but what I would also say is that those mood changes can happen at other times. They cannot be explained by a simple hormonal pattern. And that's why the simple hormonal explanation for PMS is not sufficient in my view. (Susan, critical expert [E6])

Similarly, when asked about the difference(s) between male and female experiences of non-sex-specific symptoms associated with PMS/PMDD, two of the three critical experts implied that the same symptoms had *fundamentally* different causal mechanisms, depending upon an individual's sex (due to the female reproductive body): 'I wouldn't agree that men can experience the same symptoms … I think menopausal women can, but I don't think men can, um, because … I think it is uniquely related to the female reproductive cycle and of the female reproductive pattern' (Zoe, critical expert [E16]).

Like the biomedical experts, these critical experts appeared to imply that the timing of premenstrual symptoms reflected (female sex) 'hormonal' *causality* rather than simply *correlation* (contrary to the available population data). Only Geraldine provided a more consistent 'psychosocial' causal argument for emotional distress and other premenstrual symptoms, regardless of sex.

> Well, I suppose there are some [premenstrual symptoms] that might be [sex-specific] but in general, I would say no. … I would often tell my students that, you know, a man and a woman wake up in the morning and experience some symptom and she thinks it's related to her menstrual cycle and he thinks … he's worried about his biology test in the afternoon … a lot of it is about attribution of the symptoms. (Geraldine, critical expert [E16])

The biomedical positioning of the female sex hormones as the main cause of debilitating premenstrual symptoms also clearly influenced the patients' descriptions of why such symptoms occur. Two-thirds of the patient group positioned premenstrual symptoms as entirely 'biological' in nature, with all but one of them attributing direct causality to 'hormones'. These findings were in line with previous research that has found that cisgender women (especially those of reproductive age) tend to internalise irritability or distress, and attribute it to their 'hormones' rather than external stressors.[6]

> Yeah, I definitely believe it's, it's related to the rise and fall, the natural rise and fall of the reproductive hormones, oestrogen and progesterone. (Helen, patient [P15])

> I definitely get diarrhoea, whereas other women don't, and that's apparently to do with the amount of hormones that are in your body. (Alice, patient [P15])

Gendered perspectives, symptoms and treatments

Chapters 4 and 5 have already mentioned participant discourses that prioritised certain premenstrual symptoms over others, suggestive of the influence of gender myths (exemplified by the PMS stereotype). Here I highlight some other ways in which the different participant groups used gendered discourses when describing PMS.

The PMS stereotype (that is, gender myths) as perpetuated by men

Two biomedical experts and seven patients implied that the PMS stereotype was often perpetuated by boys and men, especially within the context of school or the workplace. This is in line with critical research, which suggests that the PMS stereotype/gender myth exists to undermine women's political position, hence it is most often invoked in relation to women's authority, productivity or abilities in the workplace.[7]

> Like how male pilots would say they didn't want to ever have a female co-pilot because they couldn't trust her during the premenstrual phase. (Celia, biomedical expert [E8])

> Like for example, at work, if a female's moody they'll [male colleagues] be like 'Oh, I think she's on, do you know what I'm sayin'? And you're just thinking, 'OK, you just pissed me off now'. (Noor, patient [P19])

Attributing the PMS stereotype discourse to men and boys was also apparent in participant accounts of how they first heard about PMS. A quarter of the patients, plus one male biomedical expert, explicitly described how they first heard about (stereotypical) PMS from male family members, or, in one instance, a teacher.

Gemma: For me, it was my brother … 'You're acting that way cos you're on yer period!'
Faith: Oh, they always love that.
Gemma: They LOVE THAT! And he was the first person that said it to me. (Faith and Gemma, patients [P12])

So yeah, it was the t-shirt, my gym, my cis male gym teacher who had a t-shirt … that said, 'PMS' and something about a 'mad cow'. (Ria, patient [P12])

A possible sex/gender difference in the expert participant discourses was also identified in the interview data. As briefly mentioned in Chapter 4, just over a third of the biomedical expert group repeatedly referred to 'pure' or 'core' PMS/PMDD, relating to severe cyclical *mood* changes that only occur during the luteal phase.

[T]here's the purest of the pure PMS, a core PMS … and then there's the ones with an underlying psychological problem where it gets worse. (Chris, biomedical expert [E8])

[A]nd I think there probably is a pure form of PMDD, but I also think there's probably a lot of people that have something else, that's bubbling away, that's exacerbated premenstrually. (John, biomedical expert [E14])

Interestingly, this subgroup was comprised of all four of the male biomedical experts interviewed (a psychiatrist, a pharmacologist, a gynaecologist and an epidemiologist) but only two of the eight female biomedical experts (both of whom worked with these men). While the very small sample size prevents generalisation, this finding could indicate that the male biomedical experts were perhaps more likely to position negative mood change as *intrinsic* to premenstrual experiences, contrary to the available population data.[8]

While further research would be required to confirm (or reject) this possible discursive 'sex difference' within the expert group, there is a highly plausible explanation for it. Since male biomedical experts lack embodied experience of the menstrual cycle, they may be more susceptible to uncritical acceptance of gender myths and the PMS stereotype, which would only be reinforced by patient claims that 'all women experience PMS' and the specific subset of mood-related female patients that they encounter in clinical practice (discussed in the previous chapter).

In fact, one of these male biomedical experts even implied that premenstrual symptoms were akin to the sexual behavioural changes associated with *oestrus* (conspicuous ovulation) in other female mammals. '[T]he rudiment here is probably the oestrus cyclicity that you see also in various other species in terms of sexual behaviour and other stuff that is a behaviour change associated with the oestrus cycle. I think that this [PMS/PMDD] is a reminiscence of that in other species' (Andrew, biomedical expert [E6]). This erroneous yet persistent (sometimes demonstrably sexist[9]) comparison confuses ovulation with menstruation and assumes that premenstrual symptoms reflect pro-reproductive behaviours when, in fact, their timing typically correlates more directly with spontaneous decidualisation and menstruation, which are (when periods occur) abortifacient processes. It also implies that female behaviour/emotional expression is predominantly 'biological' in origin, thus effectively removing human agency and positioning severe cyclical symptoms, such as suicidal ideation or abdominal pain, as 'natural' rather than indicative of extreme distress (in response to traumatic experiences) and/or an underlying health condition.

Gendered symptoms and treatments

As mentioned in the previous chapter, the most common premenstrual symptoms described by the clinical and critical expert experts (combined) and the patients formed near identical lists to that derived from a good quality PMS population study (for example, Table 5.1).[10] An examination of the *differences*, however, revealed some fascinating nuances. For instance, in keeping with their tendency to focus on emotional distress, the experts overemphasised three negative mood changes (depression, anxiety and suicidal ideation) in their descriptions of the most common PMS symptoms (Table 6.1). They also mentioned a couple of additional mood-related symptoms ('tearfulness' and 'increased emotional awareness') not included in the population study list (Table 6.1).

In fact, contrary to the population data, nearly two-thirds of the patients and a quarter of the experts mentioned 'tearfulness' as a common premenstrual symptom (Table 6.1). It is worth noting, however, that several of these descriptions positioned it as 'positive' and equally likely to be triggered by joyful or pleasantly 'moving' events or experiences than by sad, irritating or stressful ones.

> So I actually like the fact that I feel more ... I just think it's a beautiful thing. Like, I like the fact that I cry. (Gemma, patient [P23])

Table 6.1: Additional and overemphasised symptoms mentioned by the experts and patients, in comparison with population data derived from Dennerstein et al (2011)

	All experts	Patients
Relatively over-emphasised symptoms	Depression Anxiety/tension Hopelessness/suicidal Loss of concentration Sleep disturbance	Appetite changes Temporary weight gain Skin changes
Additional symptoms (not listed in the population data)	Tearfulness Dizziness Increased emotional awareness	Bowel changes Tearfulness Libido changes Physical weakness Temperature changes Bleeding/spotting Cleaning

> I can watch someone singing and I'm like [indicates tears] it's just the power or the beauty of how they sang. … I feel like I can actually cry. (Faith, patient [P23])

This suggests that this type of (premenstrual) 'tearfulness' might need to be differentiated from the type of crying indicative of underlying depression or anxiety.[11] The fact that it was still labelled as a 'symptom' rather than a non-pathological, neutral or even positive change by these participants may reflect the way in which crying in general is discursively positioned as a (feminine) debility, rather than healthy human emotional expression.[12]

A different kind of gender myth appeared to influence the patients' symptom list. Most of their relatively medicalised and additional symptoms related to concerns about body image or idealised 'feminine' attributes (for example, appetite changes, temporary weight gain, acne, physical weakness and even 'cleaning') (Table 6.1). Interestingly, in response to a specific follow-up question about 'bloating', a couple of the patients directly associated it with negative body image, suggesting that the distress caused by abdominal distention is not only physical discomfort, but also psychological distress caused by feeling (even just temporarily) 'fat'. This is in line with other studies that have found women may feel pressure to conform to an idealised 'feminine standard' and so are likely to notice and feel distressed by 'non-feminine' or body-image related changes associated with the menstrual cycle.[13]

> For me specifically, it ['bloating'] means water retention. It means [pause] uh, putting on a good few pounds, having a distended abdomen.

I get bloating around my face, I get puffy eyes, so ... it's not just bloating in the lower abdomen. To me, I feel like the Michelin Man [laugh]! Sorry, I shouldn't laugh, but I feel like a fuckin' marshmallow [laugh]! It's like, yeah, it's horrible, really horrible. (Emma, patient [P25])

[T]he term bloating is just feeling heavy, feeling fat. Yeah, I do get that ... water retention. That's the worst ... and then you weigh yourself. Oh, God! (Aisha, patient [P25])

A couple of the patients also differentiated 'bowel changes', including diarrhoea, constipation and trapped gas, from the term 'bloating' (Table 6.1). In contrast, none of the experts mentioned any bowel changes and they were also omitted from the population study list (Table 6.1). As one patient observed, this relative lack of attention paid to premenstrual bowel changes was possibly because they are not *attractive* 'feminine' experiences, whereas emotional changes better fit societal gender myths.

No one wants to address the fact that women poo, anyway, so any sort of bowel symptoms don't get any kind of attention or anything that makes women look sort of unattractive [laugh]! ... I think a lot of the sort of information out there ... focuses a lot on the emotional side of things and is a bit misleading? (Beth, patient [P19])

A gendered discourse could also be identified in the participant responses to a question relating to the treatment of PMS. Around a third of the biomedical experts and one patient (who had undergone surgery) mentioned hysterectomy and/or oophorectomy as a way to manage PMS (as opposed to PMDD or any other underlying condition). As previously noted in Chapter 4, this suggested that some of the biomedical experts used the terms PMS and PMDD somewhat interchangeably, and typically implied that 'PMS' is simply a 'less severe' form of a mental health disorder (contrary to the population data and the discrete formal biomedical definitions). Most strikingly, however, a couple of these biomedical experts positioned natural or surgical menopause as *the* 'cure' for premenstrual symptoms.

There's two cures. One is a natural cure, that's the menopause and the other cure is take out the uterus, ovaries, and cervix. (Chris, biomedical expert [E7])

So, you could have a sort of natural solution, which would be menopause or a medical solution and that'll involve the available options, um, removing the ovaries and the uterus, cervix, the whole thing. (Jo, biomedical expert [E7])

In a follow-up expert-specific question about surgical interventions for PMS/PMDD, two-thirds of the biomedical experts (but none of the critical experts) endorsed them, although most clarified that surgery was very much a 'last ditch' treatment option for severe and intractable cyclical symptoms only.

> I think for some people it's appropriate but it's at the end of the line. (John, biomedical expert [E24])

> That should be a last (long pause) ditch effort. (Laura, biomedical expert [E24])

Again, one biomedical expert positioned the removal of the female reproductive organs as a 'cure' for cyclical symptoms (in this case, epileptic seizures). This quote is very interesting because it positions the menstrual cycle as the 'cause' of the seizures, rather than a triggering factor in epilepsy.

> I've used it once for a patient who had premenstrual epileptic seizures and I cured her [smile and laugh], which was really, really rewarding both for me and, of course, for the patient. But that, I think, is the only time I've ever … [performed] an oophorectomy [for cyclical symptoms]. (Marta, biomedical expert [E24])

Regardless of the insufficient evidence base for promoting surgery as a 'cure' for severe cyclical symptoms, this treatment option is highly reminiscent of deeply problematic historical biomedical discourses regarding 'female hysteria'.[14] Tellingly, the one patient who had undergone a total hysterectomy and oophorectomy for PMDD and fibroids described how she felt under pressure from others ('unfair expectation' in line 1) to be 'like men now' (lines 2–3), as if the surgery effectively removed her femininity, which was directly equated with pathological emotionality ('emotionally sterilised' in line 2) (Excerpt 6.2).

Excerpt 6.2

1 [T]here is an unfair expectation [...] that [...] women that have had the
2 surgery should now be emotionally sterilised in a way (.) like you know (.) we should
3 be like men now? (.) haha! [laughter] [...] I resent that (.) hahaha! [laughter] [...] life
4 will still happen (.) you know (.) you're cutting out your ovaries (.) not your <u>heart</u>
5 (.) haha! [laughter].
   (Helen, patient [P26])

Interestingly, Helen also explicitly contested this gender myth, by using another (non-sex-specific) embodied metaphor for human emotionality ('heart' in line 4) and referencing external factors ('life' in line 3), which effectively exonerated the female reproductive body from being positioned (by others) as the main, or sole, *cause* of her emotional distress.

Exaggerating the premenstrual problem

In contrast to the diagnostic criteria for PMDD, the current definition of PMS includes 'any' moderate–severe symptoms that occur after ovulation and resolve before or during menstruation.[15] The experts were asked how they felt about this uniquely 'open' biomedical definition. Only three biomedical experts fully endorsed it. Most experts (seven of the biomedical experts and two critical experts), indicated a somewhat ambivalent attitude, mainly due to its lack of symptom specificity. They still, however, positioned the current definition as useful in that it is 'inclusive' in terms of recognising a wide range of patient experiences. '[P]eople talk about a range, a large range of things. So, then you've really got to look at, well, what are the most prevalent of the symptoms?' (Sarah, biomedical expert [E18]). Crucially, this discourse appeared to relate to the shortcomings of the current diagnostic criteria for PMDD. Two experts (a biomedical expert and a critical expert) valued the 'any' symptoms definition because it meant that no severely debilitated patient would be turned away from treatment simply because they did not meet the (arbitrary) five-symptom minimum threshold required for a PMDD diagnosis (previously discussed in Chapter 5).

> I think it's unfair to restrict treatment to people who fulfil a group of criteria that one bunch of people have decided is correct and not to another group of people who are suffering. (John, biomedical expert [E18])

> If they say 'I've got PMS' and then they're given a standardised symptom checklist and they don't have, you know, X number of criteria on the checklist … and then we dismiss all of those women … if that's happening clinically for women who feel that they have PMS severe enough to need help, then I think that's appalling. (Susan, critical expert [E18])

Four of the biomedical experts positioned the lack of symptom specificity in the current PMS definition as a *concession* to certain members of the decision-making group, that is, that it was 'inclusive' of different professional viewpoints. They implied that 'the gynaecologists' felt that the positioning of PMDD as a mental health disorder might obscure patient experiences of debilitating physical symptoms, or perhaps even remove PMS and PMDD from the purview of gynaecology altogether. This issue of disciplinary

Table 6.2: The 17 core symptoms described by the participant groups and included in the DSM criteria for PMDD

1. Abdominal/uterine pain	10. Tension/anxiety
2. Irritability/anger	**11. Hopelessness (suicidal ideation)**
3. Digestive changes: bloating, constipation, diarrhoea	12. Appetite changes
4. Joint, back, muscle pain	13. Social withdrawal
5. Breast pain	14. Weight gain/water retention
6. Fatigue	15. Restlessness
7. Headache	16. Skin changes
8. Mood swings	17. Sleep disturbance
9. Low mood/depression	

ownership reveals the way in which the diagnostic criteria for PMS (and PMDD) were openly presented as pragmatic rather than evidence-based 'scientific' descriptions.

> [T]hat was the strong opinion from our friends in gynaecology. So, if I had written those papers myself, that would not have been my, my understanding of the situation. I'm more in the camp that want to divide these [PMS and PMDD] into different syndromes but what we said, I think, was a typical consensus group compromise that each and every symptom may qualify for PMS. (Andrew, biomedical expert [E18])

Only two of the biomedical experts and one critical expert positioned the current PMS definition as problematic since it effectively medicalised all premenstrual changes (implying that the healthy functioning of the female reproductive body is pathological). 'I think that's a bit woolly ... I think virtually all women, I mean, me included, will have had some sort of premenstrual issues ... but it's not catastrophic, it's not impacting on day-to-day living. I don't think it's reasonable to include that in a diagnostic category' (Jo, biomedical expert [E18]).

It was very interesting, therefore, to find that when asked to name the 'most common premenstrual symptoms', the expert and patient participant groups provided almost identical lists (see Chapter 5, Tables 5.2 and 5.4). What is more, these lists were also virtually identical to one derived from a large population study,[16] which was based on the diagnostic criteria for PMDD. Indeed, if the symptom synonyms found in the population list are conflated (that is, bloating/constipation, anger/irritability, tension/anxiety and water retention/temporary weight gain), the three lists are found to contain the same 17 premenstrual changes, of which only two (highlighted in bold) may be specific to PMDD (Table 6.2).

It thus appears that the most common premenstrual changes are not nearly so difficult to identify as implied by the current 'any symptom' PMS definition. What is more, they are nearly all already listed in the diagnostic criteria for PMDD. This suggests that the real issue may lie in the inclusion of non-pathological physical changes within the diagnostic criteria for PMDD, making it unnecessarily difficult to differentiate a psychiatric condition/ severe emotional distress from healthy premenstrual experiences.

To infinity and beyond; estimating the number of premenstrual symptoms

The 'any symptom' definition of PMS also implies a high number of potential symptoms or, at least, too many to list. Indeed, when asked to estimate the number of premenstrual symptoms, half of the biomedical experts provided estimates over 100, including two estimates of over 200 symptoms, and even one mention of 'infinity'.

> Over 200 [symptoms] have been described (pause). … That's why they [the expert group defining PMS] didn't set, in their definition, [any] criteria. They said that you don't have to have particular symptoms because there are so many. (Anne, biomedical expert [E9])

> We did a Delphi thing [a group consensus approach] and … we decided that … any [cyclical] symptom, physical or psychological [would count as PMS], and so it could be infinity, OK? (Chris, biomedical expert [E9])

Strikingly, all but one of the biomedical experts later claimed to *exclude* any symptoms caused by the premenstrual exacerbation (PME) of an underlying condition, when asked about this in a follow-up question. 'No, I think that they have to be differentiated … I mean you can have an underlying medical condition and PMS/PMDD, but I wouldn't say that the exacerbation of one of these conditions premenstrually is part of PMS, no' (Celia, biomedical expert [E14]).

Half of the biomedical experts thus implied that there were more than 100 premenstrual symptoms *in addition to* those associated with the cyclical worsening of underlying conditions. This strongly suggested that this discourse stems from influential (albeit inaccurate) biomedical sources such as Dalton[17] who cited 'over 100 premenstrual symptoms' (although the vast majority of these related to the exacerbation of underlying conditions), or more recently in 1994, Budeiri and colleagues[18] who listed 'over 150 premenstrual symptoms' but included several dozen symptom synonyms. Indeed, one of the biomedical experts directly referenced Dalton when making his estimate: 'Well, Katharina Dalton, if you have read her? She describes ... 150 symptoms' (Thomas, biomedical expert [E9]).

The three critical experts again appeared to be 'quoting' biomedical discourses in response to this question. However, only Susan provided a high estimate of 'hundreds' of possible premenstrual symptoms: 'There are multiple symptoms ... it's not like there's a standard where we can say "There are only 36", there may be hundreds?' (Susan, critical expert [E9]). In contrast, Geraldine critiqued the exaggerated estimates coming from biomedical/popular sources and Zoe provided a much lower estimate of 'around 20 symptoms' based on those listed in 'standard diagnostic clinical tools'. This suggested that the group as a whole was perhaps less likely than the biomedical experts to imply that there were 'too many' premenstrual symptoms to list (in PMS diagnostic criteria).

Well, I don't know. In my understanding, I can't give you a number, but it's a lot fewer than 130. I can tell you that! [Laugh] Some of them are just you know, things that people made up. (Geraldine, critical expert [E9])

Diagnostically, if we go through, you know, standard diagnostic clinical tools ... it's probably around 20 symptoms that generally would ... tend to be clustered around PMS. (Zoe, critical expert [E9])

Considering that the patients typically included 'all' premenstrual changes in their descriptions of PMS (including those that may technically count as PME), it is interesting to note that they were far less likely than the biomedical experts to grossly overestimate the number of possible premenstrual symptoms. When asked the same question, half of the group provided estimates below 30 symptoms.

Ten maybe? Genuinely no clue. (Dani, patient [P22])

Symptoms, oh, gosh! Over 20? (Aisha, patient [P22])

You know, I think around 30? (Emma, patient [P22])

Interestingly, the top three estimates came from patients with healthcare or PMS research experience, further supporting the idea that the tendency to highly exaggerate the number of premenstrual symptoms is informed by biomedical, rather than societal, PMS discourses.

It's probably loads! I think several tens, so 50 to 100? (Beth, patient and GP [P22])

I think there are 100, 200 some recorded? (Helen, patient and PMDD network founder [P22])

Exaggeration as legitimisation; estimating the population prevalence of PMS

When asked 'how common' PMS is, the average patient and expert participant group responses reflected their different definitions of PMS as either 'all' premenstrual change or 'moderate to severe mood changes/emotional distress'. For instance, the average biomedical expert estimate was 25 per cent.

Most women may identify symptoms, but a moderate to severe problem with PMS may be around 20 per cent. (Barbara, biomedical expert [E5])

It's a lot more common than I think we, we had previously thought. I mean, it might be 25 per cent of women will have some element of PMS. (Jo, biomedical expert [E5])

The critical experts were more likely to state how difficult it was to differentiate between typical premenstrual changes and those that actually disrupt daily activities (as stipulated in the formal biomedical definition of PMS). They were, therefore, more likely to describe a range of potential prevalence rates, dependent upon the diagnostic criteria used in population studies.

It's not that simple ... some studies say like 95 per cent of women get some sort of premenstrual change, but that can be quite minor. It might not be noticeable. ... There's some studies that say about 30 per cent of women get moderate changes and then this 5 to 8 per cent get severe changes. It depends on where you draw the line in terms of what PMS is. (Susan, critical expert [E5])

As mentioned in Chapter 5, the patients' estimates were very high, in line with their definition of PMS as referring to 'all' premenstrual change. The average patient population prevalence estimate was around 90 per cent (ranging from 70 to 100 per cent).

I would say that it happens in anybody that menstruates. I will say that. Yeah. (Ria, patient [P14])

I'd probably guess that about 75 per cent of women get PMS, but I've no idea, really. (Beth, patient [P14])

When compared with good quality population data, however, most participants overestimated PMS (and PMDD) population prevalence figures (Figure 6.1). Prospective population studies that incorporate some form of symptom severity measure provide more 'robust' PMS epidemiological data. Mallia's systematic review of four such PMS/PMDD studies[19] found PMS prevalence to be just 2.4 per cent to 8 per cent of the menstruating population (and PMDD prevalence to be 1.3 per cent to 2.1 per cent).[20] Only one of the biomedical experts provided a comparable estimate for PMS prevalence, and they were directly involved in one of the studies mentioned.

It is worth mentioning that three-quarters of the biomedical experts provided PMS prevalence rate estimates of 20 per cent to 30 per cent, which *were* in line with the findings of 'less stringent' (that is, lacking a measure of symptom severity) *retrospective* population studies as categorised by Mallia.[21] This suggests that the biomedical experts were perhaps more familiar with these studies. Certainly, one of the biomedical experts implied that these were indeed the source of higher estimated prevalence rates. 'I think that some of the higher estimates derive from … [retrospective] interview studies … from just women reporting they have PMS. … [For instance] If you actually try to verify prospectively … almost 50 per cent or something, actually don't have PMDD' (Marta, biomedical expert [E5]).

There are, however, a few alternative explanations for the biomedical experts' tendency to overstate the size of the PMS problem. For instance, they may have selected this (somewhat verifiable) higher prevalence rate to improve their chances of securing research funding. At least, overstating

Figure 6.1: Average biomedical and patient PMS (and PMDD) population prevalence estimates, compared to robust prospective population data

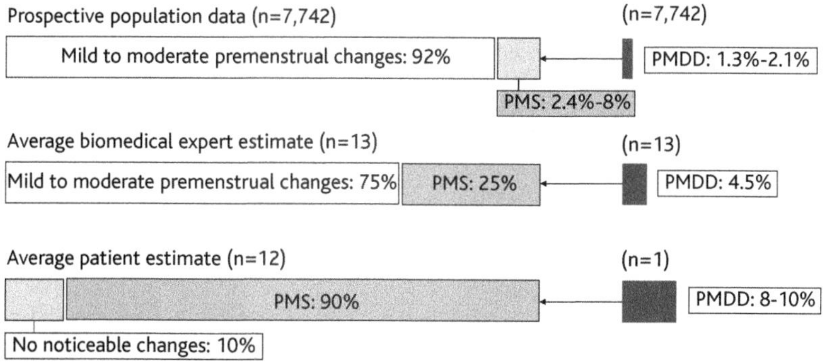

Source: Population data: Mallia (2015, pp 104–105)

population prevalence is known to be common among patient organisations (to which a quarter of the biomedical experts belong) because the larger the patient group represented, the more likely they are to access political and financial benefits, such as state or pharmaceutical research or funding.[22] The tendency to overstate PMS population prevalence could also be an attempt to *legitimise* the experiences of patients who are known to encounter societal and even clinical 'disbelief' in their symptoms. At least, some scholars have claimed that exaggeration and hyperbole (especially if the statement is essentially correct but only to a certain degree) reflect 'legitimising' rhetoric.[23] The fact that this form of exaggeration medicalises the menstrual cycle may thus be an unintentional consequence of 'good' clinical intentions, rather than simply a reflection of gender myths, such as the PMS stereotype.

As discussed in the previous chapter, half of the patients positioned PMS as 'not an illness', meaning that their high estimates of PMS prevalence do not straightforwardly equate to the exaggeration of debility in the general female population. In this way, as a group, the patients simultaneously medicalise and normalise premenstrual changes, in keeping with the snatch-22 paradox. It is also worth noting that only one of the patients provided an estimate for the prevalence of PMDD in the population (8–10 per cent) (Figure 6.1), and so this single estimate cannot be taken to reflect a general tendency towards exaggeration within the patient group.

Chapter summary

The female reproductive body was consistently positioned as the main, if not sole, cause of cyclical symptoms, with most participants implying that fluctuations in the (female sex) hormones were a causal rather than simply correlated factor in premenstrual symptoms. This suggested that the PMS stereotype/gender myth positioning women (especially their emotions) as controlled by their bodies in a way that men are not, is surprisingly powerful, in that it persists within biomedical discourses even in the face of substantial contradictory data.

What is more, even those who contest biomedical definitions of PMS/PMDD, such as the critical experts, appeared to relatively uncritically accept the idea that it was the female sex hormones that play the 'biological' role in the biopsychosocial causes of premenstrual symptoms. The patients also attributed causality to their hormones, but this is to be expected given the pervasive nature of biomedical and societal portrayals of PMS.

Several participant discourses implied that the PMS stereotype is (most) often believed/perpetuated by cisgender men. This was also reflected in the possible 'sex difference' found in the biomedical expert descriptions of 'core' or 'pure' PMS/PMDD, referring to severe premenstrual emotional distress thought to be entirely caused by hormonal fluctuations, rather than an underlying condition such as depression and/or anxiety. Gender norms also seem to have influenced the patients' discursive prioritisation of (feminine) body image-related premenstrual changes, even though such changes are not typically severe.

A potentially valuable finding of this study was that the biomedical experts may have struggled to define PMS, due to the inclusion of physical premenstrual changes in the diagnostic criteria for PMDD. This situation appears to have been caused by pragmatic rather than scientific factors, such as the need to formally recognise premenstrually suicidal individuals who do not meet the minimum number of criteria required for a diagnosis of PMDD, and to address the concerns of 'the gynaecologists' who were perhaps more aware of patients with severe physical symptoms. Unfortunately, defining PMDD in this way has made it unnecessarily difficult to differentiate it from healthy premenstrual changes.

Finally, participant tendencies to exaggerate the number of potential premenstrual symptoms, and the population prevalence of PMS/PMDD, were identified, which further implied that the female reproductive body is inherently pathological. The biomedical experts were most likely to *highly* exaggerate the number of potential premenstrual symptoms, suggesting that a couple of influential biomedical publications are the likely source of this discourse. Importantly, both sources include symptoms associated with premenstrually exacerbated conditions and several synonyms for essentially the same experiences.

The patients provided the largest average estimates for PMS population prevalence, but as previously discussed in Chapter 5, half of the group also positioned PMS as 'not an illness', which partly mitigated the implication that the female body was inherently debilitating. The biomedical expert and critical expert groups tended to cite PMS population prevalence rates typically found in less stringently defined retrospective population studies. This could also be explained by a perceived need to exaggerate the impact of PMS/PMDD to attract resources for awareness-raising and research purposes, or even to 'legitimise' the experiences of PMS/PMDD patients, known to be subject to societal and clinical disbelief.

In short, participant discourses were not based on the available data regarding the likely cause(s) of premenstrual changes or debilitating cyclic symptoms. Instead, they appeared to reflect and reproduce a key gender myth: the 'femininity as debility' myth that positions the female (reproductive) body as inherently pathological/inferior (Figure 6.2).

Figure 6.2: Positioning the female (reproductive) body as pathological

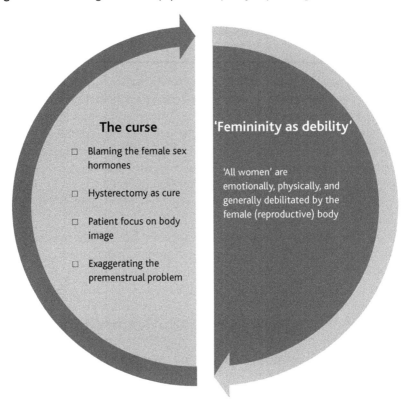

The curse

☐ Blaming the female sex hormones

☐ Hysterectomy as cure

☐ Patient focus on body image

☐ Exaggerating the premenstrual problem

'Femininity as debility'

'All women' are emotionally, physically, and generally debilitated by the female (reproductive) body

---

Box 6.1: The curse: why this matters

Science

It is bad scientific practice to disregard decades of negative findings – in this case regarding the hypothesised 'causal' role of the female sex hormones in healthy premenstrual changes, PMS and the cyclic triggering/worsening of underlying conditions/distress. Rather than accepting this data and moving on to more evidence-based theories, biomedical PMS research has instead been influenced by, and reproduces, the 'femininity as debility' gender myth. Similarly, the unscientific inclusion of typical premenstrual changes in the diagnostic criteria for PMDD appears to have unnecessarily conflated healthy physiology with a serious and potentially fatal psychiatric disorder.

Clinical practice

The biomedical PMS research focus on the female sex hormones has obscured alternative causal theories and associated treatment options for problematic cyclic symptoms. This will have undoubtedly contributed to poor patient outcomes.

Society

As nicely illustrated by the patients and critical experts, the biomedical perpetuation of the 'femininity as debility' gender myth is also reproduced within wider society. Lacking alternative biological discourses, we are forced to label our healthy experiences with a biomedical term (PMS) and to (understandably) assume that there must be something in the idea that it is our 'hormones' that cause physical and emotional distress. This contributes to the super problematic and unhelpful belief that male and female bodies and minds are *fundamentally* different things (that is, way beyond a few small genetic or physiological differences). Pain is pain and it is generally caused by the same things, regardless of your sex or gender: inflammation and/or emotionally distressing experiences. The female sex hormones are not pathological substances.

Personal

I think it is time we realised that all humans are mainly the same. We are the same species. We are not from different planets. No one population group is biologically superior or inferior. All of us experience emotional distress under certain circumstances. In fact, all the same things that make kids cry make us distressed, too: physical pain, tiredness, fear, hunger/thirst, extreme noise/shock/temperatures, social neglect/ isolation, or other people being mean or annoying. If there is a female prevalence of emotional distress (which is not for certain), it could just be that, on average, we have more distressing lives. Let us do something about that, instead of blaming the female body.

Black box: the unknown/mysterious female reproductive body

This chapter examines the way in which participants appeared limited in their ability to describe healthy (pre)menstrual physiology and experiences. This issue seemed to affect both expert and lay definitions of Premenstrual Syndrome (PMS), in that if one cannot describe the purpose or functions of the menstrual cycle, then it is more difficult to accurately differentiate healthy from problematic experiences. Of particular interest were the factors that enabled this situation to persist, given that good quality data concerning the purpose and function of the healthy menstrual cycle *do* exist.

The patients were clearly subject to different types of constraints than the experts. The first section examines how and why the patients described a straightforward 'lack of knowledge' regarding the menstrual cycle, whereas the following two sections look at the experts' apparent omission of its purpose and healthy functioning. The first of these expert-specific sections examines the way in which they tended to reduce the menstrual cycle to (female sex) hormonal changes only, omitting additional physiological processes involved in ovulation, spontaneous decidualisation and menstruation. It is argued that this reduction may contribute to the group's tendency to conflate symptom correlation with 'hormonal' causation and to position contradictory data as due to the 'mysterious' female reproductive system, rather than alternative physiological explanations. The third section describes some of the material and structural factors within clinical research and practice, which seemed to further obscure healthy menstrual physiology in the expert accounts of PMS.

Ignorance is not bliss

Throughout the interview data, expressions of 'not knowing' were so numerous that I quickly identified them as a major discursive theme. The frequency with which any individual expressed uncertainty varied a lot but, on average, the patients described a 'lack of knowledge' more often than the experts. For instance, in response to a question about the purpose of menstruation, half of the patients indicated that they 'did not know' why they had periods.

> Preparation for childbirth is the only thing I was told, the only thing I know? Still don't understand, fully. Honestly, it's really weird but I just don't? (Gemma, patient [P7])

(Pause) I guess it's for (pause) um, it's just the way our body kind of, I don't know? (Pause) It's like, it's preparing us for birth type of thing, more I think? (Aisha, patient [P7])

These expressions of uncertainty did not, however, prevent the patients from also providing *possible* explanations. For instance, two-thirds of the patients (including Beth, who is also a GP) described menstruation as a process that 'helps to prepare (the womb) for pregnancy'.

[Long pause] Erm, well they occur because human women are … fertile all the time, so in the event of not becoming pregnant … that sort of preparation and building up of the womb lining to prepare for pregnancy has to come away. (Beth, patient and GP [P7])

To get your womb ready for a baby and then it doesn't come and so the lining basically sheds and gets ready for the next month. (Dani, patient [P7])

As outlined in the first part of this book, menstruation is actually an abortifacient process, which evolved to protect us from potentially unsuccessful, costly or even fatal pregnancies.[1] This suggests that the patients' understanding of their bodies is influenced by far more accessible societal gender norms and discourses that position them as inherently 'for' conceiving, gestating and having babies.[2]

The associated idea that the womb lining *needs* to be shed 'if not pregnant' suggests that menstruation is a form of 'cleansing'. Indeed, the remaining third of the patient group described periods as 'the removal of toxins' or other imagined harmful entities, including the unfertilised ovum. In fact, the fifth most common metaphor found in the participant descriptions of PMS related to 'toxicity/dirtiness' and it was *exclusively* used by patients.

I think periods occur as part of a natural cycle … a natural way to allow our eggs to leave the body, um, because if they stayed in there they would probably cause harm [laugh]? (Kathleen, patient [P7])

For me, physically, it's a detox process. So, the period is a form of our body detoxing. (Ria, patient [P7])

Menstrual fluid is not pathological. While the positioning of menstruation as a form of 'excretion' or 'waste management' is an understandable misconception given the excretory functions of the anus and urethra (situated either side of the vaginal opening) and the appearance (and staining properties) of menstrual fluid, this discourse is also likely to be

Table 7.1: Results of an NVivo text frequency query regarding 'dirty/toxic' metaphors used to describe premenstrual experiences

Search terms: dirty OR impure OR unclean OR toxi* OR disgust* OR clean* OR purif*	
Participant (religious affiliation)	Text frequency
Ria, patient (Sikhism)	9
Dani, patient (Judaism)	7
Gemma, patient (Christianity)	6
Mala, patient (Islam)	4
Kathleen, patient (Christianity)	1
Total:	27

influenced by persistent societal and religious depictions of menstruation as (physically, spiritually and morally) 'dirty' or 'dangerous'.[3] Interestingly, all the patients using this type of metaphor were affiliated with a major religion (Table 7.1). Religious affiliation did not appear to otherwise affect participant descriptions of, or attitudes towards, PMS.

Half of the patients were also explicitly unsure when it came to describing why they thought premenstrual symptoms occur. 'Um (pause) I'm not sure, to be honest. I, I, I'm assuming that it is down to the body getting ready for the period? And maybe a slight shift in a hormonal balance [shaking head]? That's what I would think. Um, why that would affect mood, I'm not sure?' (Kathleen, patient [P15]). All but one of the patients, however, still went on to mention 'hormones' as a probable causal factor in premenstrual symptoms, further implying that this inaccurate stereotypical (and biomedical) PMS discourse is the most accessible explanation available to patients. 'I don't actually know. I think it has something to do with spiking of hormones? But I could have just completely made that up, I don't know!' (Dani, patient [P15]). The patient responses, thus, suggested that a lack of access to evidence-based discourses allows (indeed, promotes) the use of far more accessible ones and, thus, the perpetuation of societal gender myths.

What you don't know may hurt you

Interestingly, one of the patient responses illustrated the way in which increased knowledge of healthy premenstrual experiences could alleviate concern that changes are unusual, a possible problem ('strange' and 'weird' in line 3), or perhaps even irrational phenomena ('crazy' in line 2) (Excerpt 7.1). This suggests that the lack of decent menstrual education (globally) may contribute to the positioning of cyclical changes as inherently negative, pathological and/or psychological in origin and experience (Excerpt 7.1).

Excerpt 7.1

1 Gemma: I know it's TMI [Too Much Information] (.) I tell you I go [to the] toilet
2 like proper (.) it's crazy (.) like (.) for an hour I'll just be on the toilet (.) so I
3 think that that's (.) that's so <u>weird</u> [laugh] (.) I find it so <u>strange</u> [...] and then I'll
4 be fine
5 Interviewer: [...] Constipation followed by diarrhoea? [...] that's actually <u>extremely</u>
6 common-
7 Gemma: Oh (.) it makes me feel better that it's common [laugh]! (P11)

Additionally, a couple of the patients (both of whom had been formally diagnosed with Premenstrual Dysphoric Disorder [PMDD]) implied that the limited 'biological' (that is, 'hormonal') PMS discourses available to them contributed to their distress. This suggests that knowledge about more positive cyclical experiences and the life-saving purpose of spontaneous decidualisation and periods, could potentially alleviate some of the anxiety individuals may feel about cyclical changes, in line with the findings of previous studies.[4] Both patients were responding to a question about whether periods had any religious, spiritual or otherwise symbolic meaning for them and their responses suggest that they would have welcomed *any* alternative discourse that positioned their experiences as less intractable/inevitable than the 'hormonal' explanation implies ('this is just a thing you live with' and 'it's a biological process and that's it').

> No, but I kind of wish it did. ... Yeah, I think it would have been less like 'this is just a thing you live with' and more of ... why this matters to you. I think it would have made a difference. ... So, I think, um, ascribing ... more meaning to it ... like applying a less biological meaning to it, I think would have been helpful. (Helen, patient [P8])

> For me personally, no, there's no kind of spiritual (pause) I almost wish I did (pause) relate on a deep level, but for me, it is a very pragmatic thing of (pause) it's a biological process and that's it. But maybe that's because I have a very dysfunctional relationship with mine? [Laugh]. (Emma, patient [P8])

The patients' apparent lack of knowledge is not at all surprising given that schools do not currently teach students about the purpose of periods, healthy (pre)menstrual physiology, common cyclical changes, (pre)menstrual disorders, or the cyclic triggering/exacerbation of underlying health issues.[5] Additionally, as previously discussed, the relative ease with which PMS stereotype/gender myth discourses are accessed, readily explains why the patients might use them when lacking an alternative option.

Shockingly, three-quarters of the patients indicated that they first learnt about PMS as children, from their (predominantly male) peers (that is, children, not adult teachers, parents or medical professionals), and in relation to gender myths. In fact, over half of the patients described how they first heard about PMS in situations where either they or another girl were accused of 'irrational' or 'over-emotional' behaviour.

> The first awareness I had of PMS … was that it's a thing that girls and women get and it makes them stroppy and unreasonable. [Laugh] … [I was] 11, 12 when I first became aware of that and the boys would use it as an insult, really, if they thought you were being moody. (Beth, patient [P12])

It appears that many of us first hear about premenstrual changes from little boys in the playground. Not an ideal foundation for our (reproductive) health and wellbeing!

Clinical interactions

In the UK healthcare context, patients typically present their symptoms to a general practitioner (GP) before (perhaps) being referred to a PMS clinical specialist in either Psychiatry or Gynaecology. When asked about their experiences with 'doctors' the patients thus tended to describe interactions with GPs rather than clinical PMS specialists. In response to a question about clinicians' medical knowledge and training on menstrual cycle-related health issues (P18), all 12 of the patients directly stated or implied that it was inadequate. 'No! [Laugh] Is that really bad? Sometimes I feel like I'm teaching them and then they call me an "expert patient"' (Aisha, patient [P18]). Interestingly, around half of the patients implied that this perceived 'lack of knowledge' is a contributing factor in why clinicians may dismiss or express disbelief in severe (pre)menstrual experiences.

> No, I'm afraid [laugh]. Just my own experience and also from obviously, the group that I run [a fibroids support group]. I hear it from women all the time. They're not listened to. (Kathleen, patient [P18])

> From other people that I've spoken to … I don't feel like they do. I think they dismiss it as just something got to do with hormones … and there's not really an explanation or help for it? (Mala, patient [P18])

One of the patients also happens to be a GP and her response to this question supported the patients' view that general medical training does not adequately cover premenstrual disorders, suggesting that this is indeed a structural limitation.

No [laugh] … I don't think we do. … I think PMS is sort of given a bit of an 'Oh, by the way, some women get PMS, what can you do?' type thing. … I don't think it's seen as a massively important thing to know how to manage. (Beth, patient and GP [P18])

Corroborating this assessment is the fact that *none* of the five patients who sought medical advice for their severe cyclic symptoms were asked to prospectively track them over time. This included Helen, whose uterus and ovaries were surgically removed as a 'cure' for (suspected) PMDD: 'Never. Never once. Not even after I was diagnosed [with PMDD] was I ever asked to track my cycle. That was something I took upon myself after connecting with others with the disorder and … learning more on my own independently' (Helen, patient [P17]).

This suggests that their GPs either did not know, or feel the need, to differentiate their experiences from the cyclical exacerbation of underlying health conditions. This finding is in line with a US study that found that most doctors did not ask patients to record their symptoms over a minimum of two cycles (as stipulated in diagnostic guidelines), even when PMDD *was* suspected.[6] This is shocking given the potentially life-changing (indeed life-limiting) consequences of misdiagnosis, as described by one of the biomedical experts.

I had a patient in very recently who was told by a gynaecologist that she had PMS [PMDD]. She had had no children. She had a hysterectomy [and] both ovaries removed and then they changed the diagnosis to rapid cycling … bipolar disorder? And so, you know, she's (pause) well, she's going through a litigation process. But had that gynaecologist shown that they had gone through all the steps to make a clear diagnosis, I think there would have been less of a case to answer to. I think it's a big step to take somebody's uterus out, and ovaries, when you haven't got anything to prove your diagnosis. (Jo, biomedical expert [E17])

From the interview data alone, it was impossible to know for sure if the failure of these GPs to request prospective symptom tracking was because they lacked knowledge (of the premenstrual triggering/exacerbation of underlying conditions, in particular), or simply dismissed its value or relevance as a differential diagnostic procedure. What was clear from the patient responses, however, is that their GPs gave the impression of lacking knowledge about cyclic symptoms, and that this may have contributed to 'disbelief' in their experiences, and/or the inaccurate attribution of underlying health conditions to the menstrual cycle. This suggests that the 'snatch-22 paradox' described in Chapter 5 is partly perpetuated by *clinical* ignorance of menstrual health, especially the cyclic exacerbation of underlying health conditions.

The reduction and mystification of the menstrual cycle

While a lack of subject-specific knowledge and training readily explains why patients and GPs may struggle to describe healthy (pre)menstrual physiology, it cannot fully account for the PMS experts' apparent difficulties in doing so. Especially since, in stark contrast to the patients, two-thirds of the experts indicated that they first heard about PMS as a biomedical phenomenon (rather than a societal gender myth) during their professional training, as adults.[7]

> It was when I was a gynaecologist. I never heard of it before. (Celia, biomedical expert [E4])

> Graduate school. So, you know, in my 20s. (Geraldine, critical expert [E4])

This would imply that the experts were taught about the purpose, physiological functions and typically non-debilitating changes involved in a healthy menstrual cycle or, at the very least, have had access to such information. Yet, they all at some point expressed uncertainty when answering questions about normal premenstrual experiences. For instance, nearly half of the biomedical experts and two of the three critical experts implied that it was difficult to differentiate healthy from problematic premenstrual changes. In fact, one of the biomedical experts explicitly stated that the 'main benefit' of this study would be to help differentiate 'normal' from problematic cyclical (mood) changes: 'I would say that the main benefit you could do in this one [study] is to actually define when are actually these cyclical mood changes related to the menstrual cycle to be … considered as a condition and when are they actually to be … considered as normal?' (Thomas, biomedical expert [E17]).

Given that symptom severity ought to be a key and somewhat 'obvious' difference, why might so many of the expert group imply that differentiating healthy changes from regularly severe cyclic symptoms is tricky? The previous three chapters identified several expert discourses that likely contribute to this situation. For instance, the arbitrary prioritisation of emotional distress over far more common physical changes, the positioning of PMDD as a 'more severe' version of typical premenstrual change/PMS, and the tendency to position the 'female sex hormones' as the main *cause* of cyclical symptoms. Each of these discourses unnecessarily (and inaccurately) blur the lines between healthy female reproductive physiology and debilitating premenstrual symptoms (indicative of an underlying condition). In fact, as the rest of this section will argue, certain discourses appear to have actively limited the ability of the experts to describe (and possibly even conceptualise) more evidence-based accounts of (pre)menstrual experiences.

Equating the menstrual cycle with 'fluctuating hormones' only

One of the benefits of taking a Critical Realist approach was that it enabled and encouraged the identification of what may be *absent* in the dataset.[8] As described in Chapter 6, when asked about the cause(s) of premenstrual symptoms, *all* of the biomedical experts attributed them (directly or indirectly) to healthy fluctuations in the levels of female sex hormones, with very little mention of any other reproductive physiological processes.

> I personally believe … that it's a biological cause that is related to the hormonal variation in the blood. (Andrew, biomedical expert [E6])

> It is related to the effect that the hormones of the menstrual cycle have on neurotransmitters and some women are very sensitive to this. (Sarah, biomedical expert [E6])

In fact, throughout the interview data (approximately 200,000 words in total) terms connected to the female sex hormones were mentioned relatively more frequently by the biomedical experts, and nearly 350 times in total, whereas terms relating to other menstrual cycle-related physiological processes were used very rarely, if at all (Table 7.2).

The only exceptions were terms associated with neurotransmitters or neuroactive steroids such as serotonin, GABA or (allo)pregnanolone, which are mainly associated with low mood symptoms. Such terms were used by all but two of the biomedical experts but far less frequently than those associated with (female sex) 'hormones' (Table 7.2). 'When those hormone changes happen in susceptible women, and this possibly is where the genetic thing comes in [laugh], that affects neurotransmitters in the brain? So things like your serotonin, your GABA … it is those chemical changes, which can affect a woman's mental and physical health' (Anne, biomedical expert [E6]).

The biomedical experts and critical experts combined were twice as likely to mention water retention than the patients, but it was nearly always positioned as a symptom rather than an inflammatory process associated with the healthy functioning of the menstrual cycle, or as a potential cause of some premenstrual changes (Table 7.2).

> Women say they have a sort of extra fluid in their body. They feel almost like they're having a very mild oedema. (Marta, biomedical expert [E13])

Table 7.2: Results of NVivo text frequency queries regarding terms relating to healthy (pre)menstrual physiology

NVivo search term	Patients (n=12) Frequency and (% of total)	Biomedical experts (n=13) Frequency and (% of total)	Critical experts (n=3) Frequency and (% of total)	Total
	(n=11)	(n=13)	(n=3)	
Hormon* OR Oestr* OR Progest* OR steroid	103 (30%)	220 (63%)	25 (7%)	348
GABA OR neuro* OR serotonin OR *pregnanolone	(n= 1) 2 (5%)	(n=11) 36 (90%)	(n=1) 2 (5%)	40
	(n=0)	(n=0)	(n=0)	
Inflamm* OR prostaglandin* OR cytokine* OR immune OR leukocyte OR interleukin OR protein OR prolactin OR killer OR neutrophil	0	0	0	0
	(n=5)	(n=0)	(n=0)	
Iron OR anaemia OR ferritin	23 (100%)	0	0	23
	(n=9)	(n=5)	(n=2)	
(Water OR fluid) retention	16 (35%)	21 (47%)	8 (18%)	45
	(n=1)	(n=0)	(n=0)	
Temperature*	1 (100%)	0	0	1

> Patients tend to say they feel more gassy and they don't necessarily complain of diffused water retention but when … it was studied years ago, they did find that there is more fluid retention in the wall of the bowel and the abdominal wall. (Celia, biomedical expert [E13])

The only exceptions were two of the critical experts who mentioned the role of water retention in relation to weight gain or swollen and painful breasts. 'Yeah, so water retention definitely is one [symptom], breast sensitivity is related to that … sometimes women say weight gain, but that's probably [caused by] water retention' (Geraldine, critical expert [E10]). Similarly, iron-deficiency anaemia and body temperature change were mentioned as symptoms rather than a possible cause of premenstrual changes, but surprisingly, *only* by patients (Table 7.2). In fact, nearly half of the patient group mentioned that they had iron-deficiency anaemia, an important finding given the probable, albeit overlooked, role of iron deficiency in PMS.

'I've got … anaemia so when I was younger, that's why it [period pain] used to be more painful and my bones really used to hurt' (Noor, patient [P26]).

Surprisingly, terms relating to the inflammatory nature of the menstrual cycle were not used *at all* (Table 7.2). The experts' descriptions of PMS thus appeared to effectively reduce the menstrual cycle to 'fluctuations in sex hormones' only, rather than a range of complex (inflammatory) physiological processes affecting water retention, body temperature, iron levels and the immune system (Figure 7.1). This is despite seven interview questions being designed to prompt expert participants to reflect on (pre)menstrual physiology (see Appendix C, E6, E13, E14, E15, E16, E22 and E23).

The mystification of contradictory data

These discursive omissions are extremely important because, as discussed in the first part of this book, the second half of the menstrual cycle involves three inflammatory physiological events (ovulation, spontaneous decidualisation and menstruation). Plus, the most common premenstrual changes *exemplify* the cardinal signs of inflammation; pain, redness (blood flow changes), swelling (water retention) and heat (temperature increase). In fact, persisting with hormonal causal explanations, rather than considering the role of inflammation, appeared to have led some of the biomedical experts to position premenstrual symptoms as somewhat 'mysterious', or perhaps even 'irrational', phenomena. For example, the way in which contradictory empirical observations were positioned by one biomedical expert as 'a conundrum', rather than indicative of alternative causal mechanisms.

> There's a triggering event somewhere based on the rise and fall of sex steroids … [but] there's always a conundrum with women who are taking oral contraceptive pills, for example, who have symptoms that look very much like PMS/PMDD in timing as well, but their hormones are not … fluctuating. (Celia, biomedical expert [E6])

Similarly, John tried to account for variation in the timing of severe cyclical (mood) symptoms by implying that individuals must each have different 'sensitivities' to the female sex hormones. Again, data that appeared to contradict the 'hormonal causal mechanism' discourse were simply repositioned as evidence of some sort of mysterious hormone-related confounding factor.

> There is probably a genetic predisposition and then there is a sensitivity to hormonal changes, but I think that sensitivity is likely to differ from one person to the next. So, I think some people may be more sensitive to the progestogen increase that occurs at the time of ovulation. …

Figure 7.1: Diagram depicting the PMS biomedical experts' reduction of the menstrual cycle to 'fluctuations in sex hormones' only

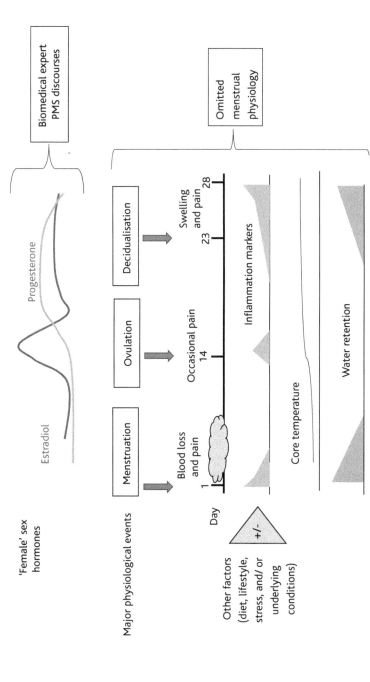

Source: Data sources informing this diagram: key events (Emera et al, 2012), inflammation levels (Salamonsen and Woolley, 1999), iron levels (Angeli et al, 2016), water retention (White et al, 2011) and body temperature (Charkoudian et al, 2017)

I think for some people it might be the drop in oestrogen that occurs [before menses]. I think for other people it's potentially something else, er, indirectly related to one or other of those things. (John, biomedical expert [E6])

Another biomedical expert even disregarded her own observations in favour of maintaining the hormonal discourse. It seems that by reducing the second half of the menstrual cycle to (higher) progesterone levels only, she had no other discursive or conceptual option other than to position her observations as 'mysterious' ('*somehow* I still think …') rather than contradictory. This also suggests that the reduction of the menstrual cycle to 'fluctuating hormones' may directly contribute to the expert tendency to conflate symptom correlation with causation.

> The symptoms only occur during the luteal phase and what characterises the luteal phase is that you have [higher] progesterone levels at that time point. But then again, it's also quite apparent that the most intense symptoms happen after the progesterone levels have declined, but somehow, I still think it's connected to progesterone. (Marta, biomedical expert [E6])

Chris, who was once involved in a trial of *Spironolactone* (a diuretic drug with anti–inflammatory properties),[9] demonstrated how his positioning of (female sex) 'hormones' as the main *causal* factor in PMS and a focus on the diuretic action of the drug (thought to reduce aldosterone hormone levels) made its effectiveness as a treatment for premenstrual symptoms seem 'illogical'. The 'hormonal' discourse thus appeared to actively prevent alternative causal mechanisms from being considered, even in the face of contradictory data. 'Well, OK, my [Spironolactone] study … showed that there were no differences in any of the hormones. No difference in aldosterone. No differences in progesterone, really. But, therefore, the logic for giving it wasn't there. But it did seem to resolve [PMS] symptoms, both psychological and particularly physical' (Chris, biomedical expert [E23]).

Prompted by these findings, I reviewed 17 of the top English-language physiology textbooks.[10] As discussed in the first part of this book, menstrual physiology beyond hormonal changes was almost completely absent from these formal biomedical accounts (Appendix A). This suggests that perhaps even the world's top PMS experts may not have had access to comprehensive menstrual physiology, even in their formal training. This was a shocking and unexpected finding, especially given that the biomedical tendency to fixate on 'hormonal changes' was first identified by Anne Walker, over 25 years ago: 'PMS has been seen as so obviously hormonally related that explicit theorising is not a requirement to research. ... This failure has resulted in poor integration of findings and inconclusive data.'[11]

Disciplinary dilemmas and other practical problems

Another benefit of conducting a Critical Realist Discourse Analysis was that it encouraged the identification of 'extra-discursive' factors.[12] These are the various embodied, material and structural conditions that can either promote or constrain certain discourses. The main embodied factors influencing patient and expert accounts of PMS (such as the types of changes and symptoms experienced or reported) have already been discussed in previous chapters. As have some of the material and structural factors relating to the experts' categorisation of debilitating physical premenstrual symptoms as something 'other' than PMS (Chapter 5), their tendency to exaggerate the population prevalence and number of symptoms of PMS (Chapter 6), and their reduction of menstrual physiology to 'hormonal changes' only (earlier in this chapter). Now we will look at some factors involved in *interdisciplinary* PMS clinical research and practice, which appeared to further obscure healthy (pre)menstrual physiology (and reproduce gender myths).

Psychiatry versus gynaecology

In response to a question about why PMS may be seen as a controversial diagnosis, three-quarters of the biomedical experts (but none of the patients or critical experts) mentioned 'interdisciplinary difficulties'. This suggests that the biomedical experts were subject to additional constraints due to the 'shared' ownership of PMS and PMDD between gynaecology and psychiatry. In fact, throughout the interview data, half of the biomedical experts directly referred to such issues as having a negative impact on the formal definition of PMS and/or PMDD.

For instance, a couple of the biomedical experts stated that the problematic inclusion of common (typically mild) physical changes in the diagnostic criteria for PMDD arose as a 'concession to the gynaecologists' involved in decision-making processes. The responsibility for doing so, however, was attributed to either 'the gynaecologists' or 'the psychiatrists', depending upon the (disciplinary) position of the speaker.

> One of the criticisms from gynaecological colleagues and academics [was] that physical symptoms should be expanded and given more weight ... that is why the [international biomedical group responsible for formally defining PMS] didn't specify any symptoms. The gynaecologists felt that the physical symptoms could be as prominent

as emotional symptoms for some women. (Fran, biomedical expert, psychiatrist [E22])

Oh I see what you mean! It [physical premenstrual change] doesn't need to be in the [diagnostic criteria for] PMDD. Well ... that'll be pragmatism on the side of the psychiatrists who said, 'Oh we'd better pay a bit of attention to the gynaecologists here' and they bunged it in! That's my real view. (Chris, biomedical expert, gynaecologist [E22])

Andrew, one of the biomedical experts who is neither a gynaecologist nor psychiatrist, directly attributed the inclusion of physical changes in the diagnostic criteria for PMDD to the (undue) influence of specific 'opinion leaders' from (UK) gynaecology. By referencing 'a good scientific argument' for the separation of PMS from PMDD (line 1) he further implied that the consensus-building process (between psychiatry and gynaecology) resulted in concession-based, rather than evidence-based, definitions of PMS and PMDD.

The others will not agree but I think there is a good scientific argument to divide these [PMS and PMDD] into ... different conditions. ... I don't think you would have any problem with psychiatrists ... to skip the eleventh item of the DSM [typically mild physical premenstrual changes], for example, and regard it as merely a mood condition. But I think it would be very difficult to convince the so-called opinion leaders ... to convince those in gynaecology, of abandoning the concept that all premenstrual symptoms are part of the same syndrome. (Andrew, biomedical expert, other [E25])

Interdisciplinary difficulties resulting in concession-based decision-making may also have contributed to the experts' tendency to position the female reproductive body as 'mysterious' or 'scientifically unknowable'. For instance, Fran described how different perspectives within the decision-making group resulted in the lack of any list of constitutive premenstrual symptoms in the formal definition of PMS, rendering the condition unusually ill-defined and, thus, somewhat 'mysterious'.

What I do remember from the original meeting is that, on purpose, they didn't specifically define what premenstrual symptoms should be included in the diagnosis [of PMS]. ... Clinicians in mental health in the group ... felt that the emotional premenstrual symptoms are what is likely to make a woman seek diagnosis and treatment, while clinicians in gynaecology seemed to think that some women present with more problematic premenstrual physical symptoms such as cramps, or breast tenderness. The committee was [therefore] not able to say that PMS comprised specific symptoms, in their view. (Fran, biomedical expert, psychiatrist [E17])

It is worth noting here that the (problematic) discursive positioning of PMDD as 'severe PMS' and the inclusion of healthy physical changes in the diagnostic criteria for PMDD, binds the two disciplines together in a way that is not the case for other exacerbated conditions. For instance, catamenial epilepsy and menstrual migraine do not 'share' disciplinary ownership between gynaecology and neurology, both are categorised as neurological complaints. In the same way that cyclical asthma is classified as a respiratory condition and not a gynaecological one. If PMDD were alternatively (and more robustly) defined as the premenstrual triggering or exacerbation of an underlying mental health condition/distress, it would no longer be categorised as a 'gynaecological' complaint, even if menstrual cycle suppression remained as a potential treatment pathway. Similarly, it would no longer make sense for psychiatry to share ownership of PMS, given that (by definition) this label would not apply to people experiencing severe cyclical mood changes.

Remarkably, one biomedical expert described how this may already be the case in the United States, where PMDD is apparently diagnosed and treated almost exclusively by psychiatrists, and the American College of Obstetrics and Gynaecology (ACOG) has publicly opposed its categorisation as a 'gynaecological' condition.

> I would say that psychiatry ... are really the experts over here [the United States] in PMDD. We created the diagnosis. You know, the DSM 5 is a psychiatric manual. ... Gynaecologists just don't want to touch it over here. ... The ACOG retracted their [PMDD] guidelines ... and they also ... refused to take any premenstrual dysphoric disorder ... presentations at their conference. (Debbie, biomedical expert; psychologist [E17])

Given these interdisciplinary difficulties, why might biomedical experts from psychiatry and gynaecology continue to support, or at least agree to, 'sharing ownership' of PMS and/or PMDD? Interestingly, Chris (a gynaecologist) later implied that there were material and structural factors (such as access to research participants and private income generation) that would be at risk if mood-related 'severe PMS'/PMDD were no longer a gynaecological concern. These factors somewhat undermined his earlier assertion that the inclusion of typically mild physical changes in the diagnostic criteria for PMDD was an arbitrary concession to, rather than in the material interests of, gynaecologists.

It's possibly better if a gynaecologist sees patients [experiencing severe cyclical emotional distress] when the GP hasn't got anywhere and the psychiatrist hasn't got anywhere. Then they should be seen by a gynaecologist ... but, that said, if you're trying to do research on it, you want them to come, in private practice, you want them to come. So, it's not quite as straightforward as that. (Chris, biomedical expert, gynaecologist [E25])

Financial factors were also cited by a psychiatrist, who suggested that part of the reason why the ownership of PMDD is shared with gynaecology (at least within the UK National Health Service) is because psychiatry cannot *afford* to treat the (exaggerated) '5 per cent of the female population' who might need treatment. (He also implies that these large numbers of PMDD patients are currently being treated by UK gynaecologists ... which is not the case either.)

In an ideal world you'd have ... psychiatrists more trained up in, as opposed to gynaecologists more trained up in [premenstrual disorders]. ... But I don't think I'd get many of my psychiatry colleagues sort of cheering that on because ... they're fire-fighting suicidal psychotic patients with a resource that's limited. They don't want to have 5 per cent of the female population who have got the severe condition that they're not currently having to treat. I don't think they want them. (John, biomedical expert, psychiatrist [E25])

Two of the critical experts and one biomedical expert mentioned that the inclusion of typically mild premenstrual changes in the DSM diagnostic criteria for PMDD, and the 'any symptom' definition of PMS, were of practical benefit to some patients (especially in the United States) who would otherwise not qualify for health insurance to cover their treatment costs. This is perhaps a more compelling rationale for the biomedical experts' tolerance of problematic definitions, and the uncomfortable 'shared ownership', of PMS/PMDD, given their expressed desire to *legitimise* patient experiences.

Let's imagine ... you have a patient who *only* feels suicidal from day 25 to 28 and never feels suicidal, um, after the period. She wouldn't fit the category [criteria] for PMDD. So, she wouldn't in America be able to claim it [insurance] from psychiatrists because (pause) ... I think that's ... partly why it was developed [PMDD] so they could say it was psychiatric? ... So, if they only had one symptom then they'd be excluded as a diagnosis with PMDD but they wouldn't for PMS. (Chris, biomedical expert [E20])

We don't set the rules on how health authorities and how medical authorities and insurance companies, um, determine access to services. ... You know, for many many women with limited access and limited resources, this [formal PMS/PMDD diagnosis] may be the only way in which they could actually receive support and services. ... If that's the only way she's going to get services or get support, then you take the label. (Zoe, critical expert [E11])

Altogether, this suggested that context-specific factors, such as the UK and US healthcare systems, competitive disciplinary agendas, plus the experts' well-intentioned desire to support patients, may have influenced the way in which premenstrual disorders are currently defined, over and above the available data. Unfortunately, as illustrated over the past four chapters, concession-based and pragmatic rather than scientific approaches appear to blur the boundaries between healthy and pathological (pre)menstrual experiences, while also reproducing problematic gender myths.

Positivism versus social constructionism

Five of the biomedical experts also described interdisciplinary difficulties between 'clinicians' and 'feminists' during their interviews. In general, the issue was presented as being that the social constructionist approach of feminist critical PMS experts implies that patient experiences (rather than merely the biomedical labels applied to them) are 'constructed' and, therefore, 'not real'.

I know that there is a concern that it [the biomedical label of PMS] stigmatises women and I would just say that most people who I have heard make that claim are not clinicians who treat patients who are suffering. (Laura, biomedical expert [E17])

There used to be a professor ... who was very critical to the concept of PMDD or PMS ... and I mean, she was claiming that this was something invented by the pharmaceutical industry to sell drugs to women (pause) and I think it's easy to have that kind of opinion when you don't meet the women. (Marta, biomedical expert [E17])

This suggested that either the social constructionist literature on PMS was not accessible to, or well understood by, the biomedical experts or perhaps that it was dismissed as 'unscientific' or 'unreasonable' as a means of deflecting criticism of (unscientific) biomedical definitions of PMS and/or PMDD. What is known is that no critical experts were invited to any of the five formal PMS definition consensus-building meetings held between 2007 and 2017. This meant that a substantial body of robust and insightful data regarding psychosocial factors in patient experiences of PMS (including problematic gender norms) was largely overlooked by those responsible for formally defining the condition.

In contrast, the critical experts appeared to be much more aware of the differences between constructionist and more positivist biomedical perspectives. All three of them described the way in which their position differed from biomedical accounts of PMS.

> I moved from a, you know, very positivist, you know, experimental viewpoint to a social constructionist 'let's dismiss it, let's deny it' [the biological aspect of premenstrual changes], [to], you know, a much more political position … where, I do acknowledge the embodied aspects of it and the hormonal aspects of it. I mean, I don't know if it's hormonal? I'm not a biomedical person. (Susan, critical expert [E26])

However, as nicely illustrated by Susan's final sentence ('I don't know if it's hormonal? I'm not a biomedical person'), the critical experts also tended to quote biomedical descriptions of (pre)menstrual physiology rather than critically engage with them. This suggests that physiological data is positioned as somehow beyond the disciplinary scope of feminist scholarship and/or critical psychology, also rendering the female reproductive body 'unknown' and somewhat 'mysterious'. While some of the inconsistencies of biomedical PMS discourses were certainly identified by the critical experts (such as the prioritisation of 'hormonal' over psychosocial explanations), deeper critical examination of the data informing such discourses, thus, appeared to be restricted by (ironically, socially constructed) disciplinary boundaries.

Chapter summary

A major underlying factor in the participant struggles to define and describe PMS was not being able to confidently describe what was 'normal' in terms of premenstrual experience. The patients typically directly expressed that they lacked knowledge about the purpose and physiology of the menstrual cycle. This was not surprising given that these topics have never been taught in schools. Importantly, there was some evidence that in lieu of evidence-based physiological explanations, the patients tended to use (and, therefore, perpetuate) highly accessible, albeit problematic, societal gender myths instead. In turn, not knowing why certain changes occur, or being limited to certain discourses, such as 'hormonal' explanations, may contribute to distress, while improved knowledge may alleviate patient concerns.

All the patients positioned GPs as 'lacking in training and knowledge about (pre)menstrual health' and several implied that this was informed by, and contributed to, societal and clinical disbelief in their experiences. This opinion was supported by the fact that none of the patients with severe symptoms were asked to track them over a couple of cycles (formally required to make a differential diagnosis between PMS and the exacerbation of an underlying health condition).

More surprisingly, half of the biomedical experts also indicated that they found it difficult to differentiate healthy from pathological (pre) menstrual experiences. The group seemed to be discursively constrained by two powerful (metaphorical) mechanisms. The reduction of the entire menstrual cycle to 'fluctuations in female sex hormones' and the (subsequent) positioning of the healthy female reproductive body as scientifically 'unknowable' or 'mysterious'. This also helped to explain why (contrary to the available data) the experts tended to conflate symptom correlation with 'hormonal' causality and were limited in their ability to consider alternative explanations for premenstrual experiences. One of the most important findings of this study was that the inflammatory nature of (pre)menstrual processes is omitted from general medical, and even specialist gynaecological physiology textbooks. This suggests that despite their formal training, biomedical and critical PMS experts may not have had access to important and relevant physiological data, as was previously assumed.

Other material and structural factors also influenced expert accounts of PMS. One of the main issues mentioned by the participants was the interdisciplinary difficulties caused by the 'shared ownership' of premenstrual disorders between (UK) gynaecology and (US) psychiatry. For instance, the international consensus-building process (principally between gynaecology and psychiatry) resulted in the formal adoption of concession-based, rather than evidence-based, biomedical definitions of PMS and PMDD. By doing so, several of the problematic discourses identified in the past four chapters became formalised, unintentionally obscuring healthy (pre) menstrual physiology and reproducing societal gender myths. Importantly, the intentions of the individuals involved in these processes may have been 'positive' – to enable further research into these conditions and to help patients access treatment or financial support – even if the consequences of such definitions are ultimately negative for patients, clinical research and practice, and women in general.

Additional 'interdisciplinary difficulties' were mentioned regarding the work of critical (feminist) experts versus biomedical descriptions of PMS and PMDD. Social constructionist accounts of (the biomedical labels) PMS and PMDD were positioned by the biomedical experts as implying that the premenstrual experiences of patients were somehow 'unreal'. It was unclear if this misinterpretation of the critical literature was due to a lack of access or understanding or functioned as a means of undermining its value. Certainly, by overlooking the psychosocial factors and gender myths influencing patient experiences, the biomedical experts' accounts of PMS as primarily a 'biological' phenomenon are inadequate. At the same time, the critical experts seemed reluctant to engage with the literature on female reproductive physiology, contributing to its positioning as mysterious and perhaps even 'beyond criticism'.

In short, participant discourses were not based on the available data regarding healthy menstrual physiology. Instead, they appeared to be informed by (and to reproduce) yet another gender myth, that of the 'mysterious female body'. This myth positions the female (reproductive) body as somehow beyond scientific knowledge and enquiry, rendering it mysterious, and perhaps even irrational (Figure 7.2).

Figure 7.2: The unknown/mysterious female reproductive body

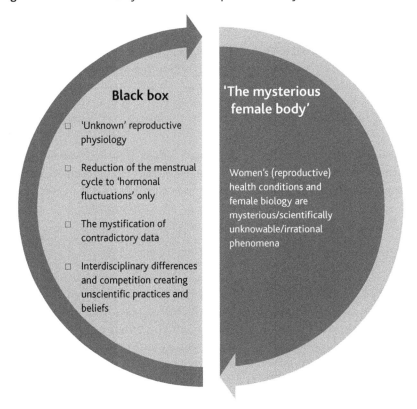

Box 7.1: Black box: why this matters

Science

The reduction and mystification of healthy menstrual physiology has severely impeded clinical research regarding PMS and the cyclic exacerbation of underlying conditions. It has obscured the likely involvement of inflammation and iron deficiency in such experiences and resulted in the positioning of confounding data, as 'mysterious' rather than 'negative'. This is an extreme case of confirmation bias, given that hormonal causal hypotheses were first put forward almost a century ago and remain unsubstantiated.

Clinical practice

I argue that it should be very easy to diagnose menstrual health and associated conditions. If a patient is not iron deficient and anti-inflammatory approaches (lifestyle, dietary or medications) have little or no impact on regularly severe cyclical symptoms, then that person most likely has an underlying condition. Imagine how much quicker this would make getting a provisional diagnosis of endometriosis, Polycystic Ovary Syndrome, heavy menstrual bleeding, PMDD, fibroids or migraine.

Similarly, understanding the inflammatory physiology of the healthy menstrual cycle and how to reduce it could improve the quality of life of half the human population, on a regular basis, for an average of 40 years each!

Society

The reduction of healthy menstrual physiology to just its hormonal coordination has resulted in nearly a century of bad science, painful and distressing life experiences for a huge proportion of the population, and the perpetuation of problematic gender and race myths. Women and other oppressed groups are not biologically inferior. We are not 'hormonal', at least not any more so than any rich White cisgender men.

Personal

We all need to know that physical and emotional reactions to cyclic pain and inflammation are normal, rational and akin to the same changes all humans experience if tired, injured, hungry, in pain, ill or affected by irritating/upsetting experiences. Those of us with underlying health conditions triggered or worsened by the menstrual cycle deserve quick and effective diagnosis and care. Just because symptoms are cyclical, does not make them less severe, 'real' or worthy of treatment. Menstrual health matters!

8

Conclusion and call to action

So, what can we conclude from the themes identified in the Premenstrual Syndrome (PMS) study data and what does this mean for women's health research and practice more widely? The first section of this final chapter outlines how and why the participant descriptions of PMS reflect three key societal gender myths more than the available information regarding premenstrual experiences. The second section summarises the wider implications of these findings and makes some suggestions for improving women's health research and associated clinical practice. I end with an urgent call to action: we must improve menstrual education if we are ever to alleviate female prevalent symptoms and conditions, *and* successfully counter the myth of the hysterical/hormonal female or Other.

Bad science, but good intentions?

The adapted Critical Realist Discourse Analysis methodology (described in Chapter 3) proved to be an extremely good fit for researching this topic. It enabled the identification of several key discursive patterns and embodied, material and institutional factors influencing participant accounts of PMS. But before discussing the first research question, 'How and why are certain premenstrual changes prioritised over others in expert and patient descriptions of PMS?', it is useful to briefly discuss the findings in relation to the second research question, 'How do expert and patient descriptions of PMS compare with robust population data on premenstrual changes?'. This way, you'll get a reminder of which changes were prioritised by whom, before getting into the 'how and why' this may have been the case.

Bad science

Participants were asked a set of questions designed to elicit comparable descriptions of PMS and the type, number, population prevalence and cause(s) of symptoms associated with this label. Three discrete participant groups were clearly identifiable. The 'biomedical expert', 'critical expert' and 'patient' groups. Group discourses were then compared with the most relevant source of population data regarding premenstrual symptoms (as outlined in Chapter 3).

A major finding of this study was that *none* of the participant group descriptions of premenstrual symptoms consistently reflected the available data (Table 8.1). This strongly suggests that the participants were describing something other than what has actually been observed in the general menstruating population. In the case of the experts, this is also indicative of poor scientific method, given that biomedical and scholarly descriptions are supposed to be based on robust methodological processes and empirical data.

Surprisingly, the patient group descriptions were more in line with the findings of population studies than those of the world's top PMS experts. The patients' descriptions of symptom type (the ratio of mood to physical symptoms), number and the 'most common' premenstrual symptoms were all very close to the population study findings (Table 8.1). This is perhaps because the patients were basing their descriptions on experience rather than 'learned' discourses.

In contrast, the only expert discourse that accurately reflected the population study data (and patient accounts) concerned the 'most common' premenstrual symptoms (Table 8.1). This suggests broad agreement on this one aspect of defining PMS, contrary to the current formal PMS diagnostic guidelines that state 'any' symptom counts (discussed in Chapter 6). Four of the seven claims made by the critical expert group were explicitly 'quoted' as coming from a biomedical source rather than directly representing their social constructionist perspective (Table 8.1). This is in keeping with the finding that the group tended to do this when asked questions that were not easily addressed using psychosocial explanations alone. It also suggests that certain biomedical PMS discourses were taken up by this group in a less critical way than others.

The main research question, 'How and why are certain premenstrual changes prioritised over others', was addressed in relation to these findings. Namely, the experts' relative prioritisation of four mood changes (anxiety, depression, suicidal ideation and feeling 'out of control'), a couple of less common and typically mild changes (concentration and sleep issues) and their minimisation of cyclical pain (period pain, headache and muscle/joint pain). Similarly, the patients' prioritisation of three typically mild body image-related cyclical changes (water retention/weight gain, skin changes/acne and appetite changes) and minimisation of headache and muscle/joint pain (but not period pain).

The second major finding from my study was that the participant descriptions of PMS seemed to be influenced by, and to reproduce, three pervasive societal gender myths. Indeed, three of the four main discursive themes drawn from the interview data almost exactly corresponded with these myths: that women are inherently debilitated by the female (reproductive) body; that women (perhaps even more so if Black or of another racialised ethnicity) are biologically prone to exaggerate/imagine/invent (symptom) experiences; and that women's cyclical physiological changes (and the female reproductive body in general) are mysterious, scientifically unknowable and inherently contradictory (that is, irrational) phenomena (Figure 8.1).

Table 8.1: Comparison of the claims made in participant group descriptions of premenstrual symptoms versus the available population data

	Biomedical experts (n=13)	Critical experts (n=3)	Patients (n=12)	Population data
Ratio of mood: physical symptoms listed	✗ 2:1	✗ 1:1	✓ 1:2	1:2 (Dennerstein et al, 2011)
Most common symptoms listed	✓ 21 (Expert group lists consolidated)		✓ 22	23 (17 in common) (Dennerstein et al, 2011)
Types of symptoms emphasised or minimised in relation to population data	✗ - Four mood changes emphasised - Two behavioural changes emphasised - Three pain changes minimised (Expert group lists consolidated)	✗ - Four mood changes emphasised - Two behavioural changes emphasised - Three pain changes minimised (Expert group lists consolidated)	✗ - Three body image changes emphasised - Two pain changes minimised	(Dennerstein et al, 2011)
Estimated # premenstrual symptoms	✗ 100+	(✗) 20–'Hundreds'	✓ 25	Approx. 23 (Dennerstein et al, 2011)
Estimated PMS population prevalence	✗ 20%	(✗) 5–30%	✗ 90%	2.4–8% (Mallia, 2015)
Main biological cause cited	✗ (Female sex) hormone sensitivity	(✗) (Female sex) hormones	✗ (Female sex) hormones	Not hormonal – but is associated with higher levels of certain inflammation markers (Gold et al, 2016)
Stated relationship between PMS and PMDD	✗ PMDD as severe PMS (and vice versa)	(✗) PMDD as severe PMS	✗ PMDD as severe PMS	PMDD is likely the PME of underlying distress or mental health condition (Romans et al, 2012)

Notes: A tick indicates broad discursive alignment with the epidemiological data source, a cross indicates a substantial difference. Brackets denote a discourse explicitly 'quoted' as coming from a biomedical source.

Figure 8.1: The three societal gender myths reflected in the four main discursive themes inductively derived from the interview data

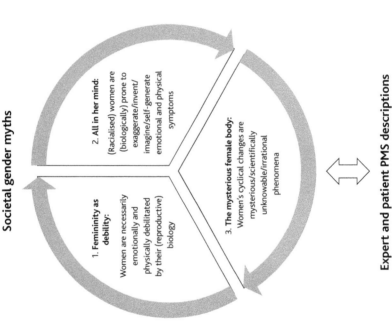

Societal gender myths

1. Femininity as debility:
Women are necessarily emotionally and physically debilitated by their (reproductive) biology

2. All in her mind:
(Racialised) women are (biologically) prone to exaggerate/invent/ imagine/self-generate emotional and physical symptoms

3. The mysterious female body:
Women's cyclical changes are mysterious/scientifically unknowable/irrational phenomena

Expert and patient PMS descriptions

Figure 8.1: The three societal gender myths reflected in the four main discursive themes inductively derived from the interview data (continued)

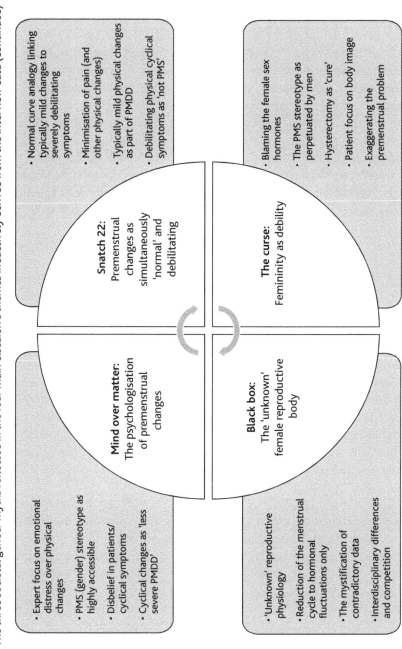

Snatch 22: Premenstrual changes as simultaneously 'normal' and debilitating

- Normal curve analogy linking typically mild changes to severely debilitating symptoms
- Minimisation of pain (and other physical changes)
- Typically mild physical changes as part of PMDD
- Debilitating physical cyclical symptoms as 'not PMS'

The curse: Femininity as debility

- Blaming the female sex hormones
- The PMS stereotype as perpetuated by men
- Hysterectomy as 'cure'
- Patient focus on body image
- Exaggerating the premenstrual problem

Mind over matter: The psychologisation of premenstrual changes

- Expert focus on emotional distress over physical changes
- PMS (gender) stereotype as highly accessible
- Disbelief in patients/cyclical symptoms
- Cyclical changes as 'less severe PMDD'

Black box: The 'unknown' female reproductive body

- 'Unknown' reproductive physiology
- Reduction of the menstrual cycle to hormonal fluctuations only
- The mystification of contradictory data
- Interdisciplinary differences and competition

Each of the three participant groups used discourses that reproduced these gender myths, but in different ways and to different extents. The discourses used by the biomedical experts appeared to be the most gendered, in that they consistently prioritised severe cyclical emotional distress/mood symptoms over more commonly experienced physical changes and minimised cyclical pain (all in her mind). They attributed premenstrual symptoms principally to the female sex hormones (despite nearly a century of research failing to find any direct causal relationship), included common physical changes in their descriptions of Premenstrual Dysphoric Disorder (PMDD), and exaggerated the number of premenstrual symptoms and their population prevalence (femininity as debility). The group also positioned premenstrual mood changes as almost entirely 'biological' in origin (rather than bio*psychosocial*), contradictory data as 'mysterious', and they reduced menstrual physiology to hormonal fluctuations only (the mysterious female body). (Appendix G provides a more comprehensive list of the various participant group discourses reproducing these gender myths.)

In comparison, the critical experts explicitly and consistently opposed the reproduction of such gender myths. However, this did not mean that they completely avoided doing so themselves. For instance, they also prioritised mood over physical changes and somewhat minimised cyclical pain (all in her mind). They largely attributed the biological component of premenstrual symptoms to the female sex hormones, and two of the group also endorsed the inclusion of common physical changes in biomedical definitions of PMDD (femininity as debility). They too, reduced menstrual physiology to just 'hormones' and two of the group endorsed the 'any symptoms' definition of PMS (the mysterious female reproductive body). Crucially, however, in many of these instances, the critical experts were explicitly 'quoting' biomedical discourses rather than necessarily *endorsing* them (see Appendix G). This suggests that the group's reproduction of gender myths was possibly due to a lack of access to any *alternative* 'biological' discourses.

The patient group also reproduced the three gender myths to a lesser extent than the biomedical expert group, but they did so in substantially different ways. For instance, the patients tended to pathologise three typically mild physical changes associated with idealised femininity (especially body image), and all cyclical changes were described as constituting 'PMS', which meant that the group's average estimated PMS population prevalence was *highly* exaggerated (femininity as debility). However, half of the group also stated that PMS is 'not an illness', which suggests that some of these medicalising discourses were due to the group's lack of access to alternative terms with which to describe different kinds of premenstrual experiences. The patients also minimised a couple of pain-related changes, and while only seven of the group had heard of PMDD, all of those that had positioned it as 'severe

PMS' (all in her mind). Finally, the group reduced menstrual physiology to 'hormonal fluctuations' but explicitly stated that they 'lacked knowledge' on this topic, and some of the group implied that cyclical changes were 'crazy', 'weird' or otherwise 'concerning' *due to* this lack of knowledge (the mysterious female body).

Good intentions

If persistent societal gender myths largely explain *why* certain premenstrual changes were prioritised over others, what explains *how* this occurred? Especially given that robust population data about the type, severity, relative prevalence and physiology of cyclical changes *is* available (at least to the PMS experts)? Another major finding of this study was that several interrelated discursive mechanisms and embodied, material or institutional extra-discursive factors seemed to actively enable or constrain the participant discourses. The main ones are listed in Table 8.2 in the order in which they were identified and discussed over the previous four chapters.

Again, the ways in which the three participant groups were influenced by these mechanisms and factors varied. The biomedical experts' descriptions were subject to all 12 of the main ones identified, the critical experts' to eight, and the patients', six (Table 8.2). This suggests that these factors played a substantial role in shaping the different participant group descriptions of PMS and perhaps the relative extent to which they reproduced gender myths. It is worth noting that these mechanisms likely interacted with, and mutually reinforced, each other. For example, the existence of a highly accessible societal PMS stereotype/gender myths plus the 'normal curve' analogy could have enabled debilitating cyclical mood symptoms (PMDD) to be positioned as a 'more severe' version of typical premenstrual change and not the cyclical exacerbation of an underlying condition/emotional distress, contrary to the available data.

It is also worth noting that the seven discursive mechanisms and extra-discursive factors affecting all participants (Table 8.2), were not intentionally employed by any individual participant or group, and that they appeared to function without the conscious awareness of the speaker. There was no indication that any of the participants were knowingly reproducing gender myths, except for when they were asked to describe the PMS stereotype. Indeed, nearly all the participants expressed the need to counter such societal beliefs during their interviews. Indeed, this was the explicit intention of the critical experts, and it can be assumed that the mainly female biomedical expert group and entirely female patient group would also have no cause to intentionally or knowingly reproduce myths that negatively impacted their own socio-political status. This suggests that much of the power of these widely used discursive mechanisms and extra-discursive factors lies in their invisibility and internalisation.

Table 8.2: The key enabling and constraining discursive mechanisms and extra-discursive factors affecting participant group descriptions of PMS

Discursive mechanisms	Participant group affected
1. Fundamental differences between biomedical, critical and patient definitions of PMS	1. All
2. The highly accessible PMS (gender) stereotype	2. All
3. The inclusion of PMDD as a discrete diagnosis (rather than the exacerbation of underlying distress) in the DSM	3. Biomedical experts
4. The inclusion of typically mild physical changes in the criteria for PMDD	4. Biomedical and critical experts
5. The use of the normal curve analogy linking typically mild to severely debilitating experiences	5. All
6. Alternative diagnostic categories and treatments for physical symptoms and 'hormonal' explanations	6. All
7. The reduction of the menstrual cycle to hormonal changes only (even in specialist textbooks!)	7. All
Extra-discursive factors	**Participant group affected**
8. The relative clinical importance of suicidal ideation over other cyclical changes	8. Biomedical experts
9. Male decision-makers and peers may believe/perpetuate PMS (gender) stereotypes	9. All
10. The tendency to highly exaggerate the number of cyclical symptoms or PMS population prevalence	10. Biomedical experts and patients
11. Lack of school/medical education in menstrual physiology and gender myths	11. All
12. The way in which clinical research and practice is funded/influenced by material interests	12. Biomedical experts

The fourth major finding of this study helps to explain how such influences can remain 'invisible', even to the world's top experts in PMS. The 'mysterious female (reproductive) body' gender myth appeared to substantially constrain the discourses available to the participant groups. For instance, the biomedical experts' reduction of menstrual physiology to 'hormonal fluctuations' is likely informed by the fact that this is how it is typically represented, even in specialist medical physiology textbooks (Appendix A). Such a major omission in the biomedical educational literature is not easily explained in scientific terms, given its obvious relevance to female reproductive health and the fact that more comprehensive physiological data about the menstrual cycle (including the role of inflammation) are available in journal articles[1] and have been in existence for several decades.[2] While it is beyond the scope of this study to come to any firm conclusion, the omission does suggest that, in line with the critical literature, biomedical PMS discourses have perhaps been reflective of gender myths more than the available data, for a very long time.

In turn, the reduction of the menstrual cycle to 'hormonal fluctuations' seemed to constrain the causal discourses available to the biomedical experts, by only enabling those involving the female sex hormones to seem plausible, despite consistently negative study findings. Indeed, such contradictory data seemed to be positioned by several biomedical experts as evidence of the 'mysterious' nature of the female reproductive system, further suggesting that biomedical PMS discourses both reflect, and *contribute* to, societal gender myths.

By 'quoting' these constrained biomedical discourses, the critical experts also unintentionally reproduced some of the same gender myths. In their case, the 'unknown female (reproductive) body' trope appeared to prevent them from critically engaging with the biological element of biomedical PMS discourses, although a reluctance to engage with biology (due to concerns about reinforcing problematic essentialist methodologies and perspectives) has been identified as an issue in feminist/critical health scholarship more widely.[3]

Finally, the patient group were much more consciously aware of their limited knowledge of menstrual physiology and appeared to reproduce gender myths mainly due to a lack of any alternative discursive options. For the patient group, it was clear that the relative ease of access to societal gender myths compared to more comprehensive physiological explanations actively constrained their discursive choices, even when they were recognised as somewhat inadequate or inappropriate. This further suggests that a lack of access to more evidence-based descriptions of premenstrual changes and disorders resulted in the unintentional and 'blind' use of discursive mechanisms that reproduce gender myths.

Crucially, the two discursive mechanisms and three extra-discursive factors of which the participants *were* (made) explicitly aware were all associated with 'good clinical intentions' (Table 8.3). For instance, the inclusion of common physical changes in the diagnostic criteria for PMDD was justified by three of the experts as 'enabling patients to access treatment', especially in the United States where private healthcare insurance only covers the treatment of conditions listed (with an associated billing code) (Table 8.3).

The fact that all five of these more 'intentional' discursive devices and extra-discursive factors were principally associated with the biomedical experts, and justified by some as a means of legitimising patient experiences or enabling access to treatment, suggests that they (somewhat ironically) were a conscious attempt to counter some of the practical issues caused by societal and clinical disbelief in the experiences of female patients (that is, the 'all in her mind' gender myth) (Table 8.3). In other words, some of the mechanisms and factors shaping the discursive reproduction of gender myths in the biomedical expert descriptions of PMS were perhaps employed to try and counter one element of them.

Table 8.3: The demonstrated intentions of the five discursive mechanisms and extra-discursive factors explicitly discussed by the participants

Discursive mechanisms discussed	Participant group affected	Demonstrated intention
2. The inclusion of PMDD as a discrete diagnosis (rather than the exacerbation of underlying distress) in the DSM	Biomedical experts	To legitimise and enable patients with cyclical rather than chronic symptoms to access treatment/healthcare insurance coverage
3. The inclusion of typically mild physical changes in the criteria for PMDD	Biomedical and critical experts	To legitimise and enable patients with debilitating cyclical symptoms (of any type) to access treatment/healthcare insurance coverage – and a political concession to 'the gynaecologists'
Extra-discursive factors discussed	**Participant group affected**	**Demonstrated intention**
8. The relative clinical importance of suicidal ideation over other cyclical changes	Biomedical experts	To try to prevent serious harm or the loss of patient lives
10. The tendency to *highly* exaggerate the number of cyclical symptoms or PMS population prevalence	Biomedical experts and patients	To legitimise patient experiences of all types of cyclical symptoms – and improve chances of securing research funding – or no alternative term for healthy changes
12. The way in which clinical research and practice is funded/influenced by material interests	Biomedical experts	To legitimise and, thus, fund research into cyclical symptoms/enable (US) patients access to healthcare insurance coverage – and enhance income and/or specialist clinical knowledge through private practice or running pharmaceutical trials

Other, less altruistic, participant explanations for the use of the same mechanisms and factors, however, alluded to material interests in the clinical 'ownership' and treatment of cyclical symptoms. For instance, the inclusion of typically mild physical symptoms in the diagnostic criteria for PMDD was described by four of the biomedical experts as a well-intentioned 'concession to the gynaecologists' (to maintain joint clinical ownership of PMDD). Thus, the fifth major finding of this study was that 'good clinical intentions' may provide a more compelling explanation for the perpetuation of unscientific biomedical definitions of PMS and PMDD than the 'material interests' previously identified in the critical PMS literature.[4] This is not to pretend that these material factors do not exist, just that the biomedical experts consistently described and demonstrated their overriding concern for their patients, or colleagues, which made it seem a more likely primary personal interest than a financial one.

So what? Key implications

My final research question was about the 'possible implications of these expert and patient descriptions of PMS on clinical, academic and societal beliefs and practices'. You will probably already be aware of some of these as they have been popping up in the 'Why this matters' boxes at the end of each chapter, but here are the five main themes again.

1. The (unintended/well-intentioned) reproduction of gender myths

Descriptions of premenstrual changes, and PMS, that are *influenced by* gender myths can also *contribute to* their perpetuation by appearing to demonstrate their 'validity' (for example, the PMS stereotype). This is perhaps especially the case for biomedical PMS discourses, which are assumed by the public to be 'scientific' and, thus, accurate and politically neutral accounts. Therefore, regardless of the good intentions of those involved in the development of formal biomedical definitions of PMS and PMDD, the consequences are ultimately negative for their patients, and women in general, if such definitions continue to reinforce gender myths.

The study also identified several key mechanisms and limiting factors that appeared to actively restrict the discursive options available to participants and, crucially, prevent them from recognising that this was the case. This suggests that certain discourses persist, despite overwhelming contradictory empirical data, due to the 'invisible' power of such factors making them seem like common-sense or pragmatic responses to acknowledged inconsistencies or problems. While this cannot fully excuse the 'bad science' demonstrated throughout the history of biomedical PMS research, it does at least help to explain why numerous highly trained and well-intentioned individuals have endorsed, or at least tolerated, unscientific practices and definitions of cyclical symptoms, despite consistent scholarly criticism.

Indeed, even those who were explicitly opposed to the reproduction of gender myths in descriptions of PMS could not help but unintentionally do so, through a lack of access to or engagement with alternative 'biological' discourses or data (possibly due to factors associated with the myth of the mysterious female body). These findings could, therefore, also be relevant for clinical and critical health research on other female-prevalent health conditions, such as irritable bowel syndrome, ME, fibroids, endometriosis, Polycystic Ovary Syndrome, perinatal depression, perimenopausal changes and various auto-immune disorders, including fibromyalgia.

2. Poor patient experiences and health outcomes

Societal and clinical disbelief in, or the dismissal of, the experiences of women in general (and especially if Black or another racialised ethnicity) was acknowledged as a substantial problem for patients by all participant groups. Unfortunately, the biomedical experts' desire to support patients by legitimising their accounts of physical cyclical symptoms through their inclusion in the Diagnostic and Statistical Manual of Mental Disorders (DSM) (thus enabling US patients to access healthcare insurance to cover treatment costs) unintentionally contributes to the very same 'all in her mind' gender myth, because common cyclical changes are now formally associated with a psychiatric disorder. This problem may have much wider implications given that clinical disbelief in, or dismissal of, the complaints of female patients is historically associated with the female reproductive body (the myth of, 'hysteria') and known to extend beyond cyclical symptoms. For instance, disbelief is a factor in the higher rates of maternal mortality for Black and other racialised women,[5] and the misdiagnosis or under-treatment of female pain,[6] including potentially fatal cardiovascular symptoms.[7]

The different perspectives of the clinical specialisms involved in defining, diagnosing and treating PMS and PMDD means that a patient experiencing cyclical symptoms may have access to different types of support, depending on the discipline of their clinician. In short, the patient experience is heavily dependent upon circumstance, rather than any consolidated biopsychosocial treatment guidelines covering both physical and mood-related cyclical symptoms. In fact, for this reason, biomedical PMS experts have previously attempted to standardise clinical practice by publishing a set of diagnostic and treatment guidelines for PMS, but they only really address severe emotional distress, that is, 'PMDD'.[8] This study's finding that severe physical cyclical symptoms are typically categorised as something 'other' than PMS and are more easily diagnosed and treated at the GP level, could be very useful in future attempts to standardise good clinical practice and improve patient outcomes for all cyclical symptoms, without unintentionally reproducing any gender myths.

3. Poor clinical training and school education

A major finding of this study was that a lack of access to, or engagement with, information about menstrual physiology plays a key role in the unintentional reproduction of gender myths in both the expert and patient descriptions of PMS. For the patients, their expressed 'lack of knowledge' about the female reproductive body was described by some as contributing to their distress and was demonstrably an enabling factor in their uptake of gender myth informed discourses. Similarly, the experts' reduction of menstrual physiology to 'hormonal fluctuations' seemed to actively constrain their ability to identify and engage with alternative causal mechanisms and be reflective of the myth of the 'mysterious' female (reproductive) body.

The wider implications of these findings relate to what is taught to all children at school. A greater public understanding of the purpose and function of the menstrual cycle could have a beneficial impact on female health, self-esteem and ability to counter and avoid the internalisation of damaging gender/racial myths. GPs (as the primary clinicians interacting with patients), gynaecologists and critical PMS scholars would also benefit from the inclusion of more comprehensive menstrual physiology in their professional training. Ideally, this would also include the way in which gender and racial myths are unintentionally reproduced in biomedical (and even critical) female health discourses.

4. The unnecessary separation of biological and psychosocial data

In keeping with Critical Realist theory in general, it was found that 'realist/ social constructionist' 'biomedical/critical' perspectives on PMS were not incompatible, nor always in opposition with each other. The biomedical and critical expert groups were simply describing slightly different elements of the same phenomenon. It was also clear that the critical experts were more engaged with biomedical discourses (being able to 'quote' them directly) than the biomedical experts were with theirs. In fact, the biomedical experts appeared to misinterpret critical 'feminist' arguments as implying that debilitating premenstrual symptoms were, in themselves, socially constructed. This suggests that it might be beneficial for biomedical and critical PMS experts to share the same definitions of typically mild (non-pathological) changes versus debilitating (pathological) cyclical symptoms (indicative of underlying conditions), to better enable the integration of 'biological' and 'psychosocial' research findings/data.

This type of tension between disciplines is unproductive and contributes to negative patient experiences and outcomes. For example, current biomedical guidelines do not mention any psychosocial factors in, or treatment options for, PMS (other than a brief mention of cognitive behavioural therapy[9]). This is despite the fact that critical work has shown that psychological and educational interventions designed to increase knowledge of, and create more positive associations with, the female reproductive body can reduce the severity of all types of cyclical symptoms.[10] Similarly, by not engaging critically with the 'biological' element of PMS, the critical psychologists seem to have overlooked the fact that hormonal explanations are not supported by the available data. These findings may have implications for research on, and the treatment options available for, all kinds of female-prevalent health conditions.

5. Inadequate research into the causes and treatment of cyclical symptoms

Finally, the experts' prioritisation of mood-related cyclical symptoms may have limited their ability to engage with alternative causal mechanisms (and associated treatment options), as well as reproducing gender myths. For instance, the biomedical experts' apparent focus on trying to isolate a distress-causing chemical may have prevented them from exploring mechanisms that would also account for psychosocial influences on physiological processes, the cyclical exacerbation of numerous underlying mental and physical health conditions, and the physiology of 'normal' premenstrual changes. Alternative, biological causal theories, such as 'inflammation', are not only more robust but also potentially less stigmatising, in that they are not sex-specific experiences.

The current definitions of PMS and PMDD make differentiating them from each other and healthy physiological changes unnecessarily difficult. This also makes the comparability and replication of clinical studies extremely difficult. Having more evidence-based definitions of cyclical changes and symptoms could, therefore, help improve the quality of clinical and academic research. Indeed, the various factors identified in this study as contributing to the reproduction of gender myths could be included in guidance for menstrual health researchers, building on existing 'good practice' research guidelines.[11]

Chapter summary

Determining what 'counts' as a premenstrual symptom is not as straightforward as one might think. Currently, it really depends on *who* you ask and their embodied, educational and socio-cultural experiences and perspectives. Individuals who self-identified as experiencing problematic cyclical symptoms (typically labelled PMS) described predominantly physical experiences, ranging from mild to severe, in line with the available data regarding the general menstruating population. Biomedical and critical experts in PMS research, however, predominantly described moderate to severe cyclical emotional distress.

Conducting a Critical Realist Discourse Analysis usefully identified several discursive and extra-discursive themes and factors that seemed to enable or constrain these participant group discourses. By comparing them with robust population data, it was possible to assess the discourses' relative explanatory power and/or (unintentional) reproduction of societal myths, such as the 'hysterical/hormonal/irrational female'. This methodology also enabled the identification of a major discursive omission in participant accounts, namely menstrual physiology beyond its hormonal coordination. While this was not unexpected in the case of the patients given the typically poor quality of menstrual education globally, it was more surprising to observe in professionally trained, highly experienced and diligent biomedical and critical researchers.

A subsequent review of school and medical textbooks found that menstrual physiology beyond hormonal changes was absent.[12] In this way, it appears that the metaphorical pairing of 'women' and 'hormones' has limited scientific and societal knowledge regarding menstrual physiology. In lieu of an alternative explanation, gender myth-informed discourses are (unintentionally) reproduced by those trying to account for, and attend to, cyclical symptoms. This is a two-way (cyclical!) interaction between societal and biomedical discourses that mutually reinforces problematic gender norms and associated discriminatory beliefs and practices, rather than a conscious or purposefully sexist or profiteering scientific agenda (even if such factors have played a part).

I argue that by integrating more comprehensive menstrual physiology, evidence-based and less 'mysterious' definitions of premenstrual and other female-prevalent symptoms are possible. In fact, systemic inflammation and/or iron deficiency offer relatively straightforward explanations for premenstrual changes, given that the luteal phase is a series of three pro-inflammatory events, which trigger regular blood loss. Systemic inflammation also provides a means by which to explain the cyclical triggering or worsening of underlying conditions, plus the way in which psychosocial factors can influence our bodies (and vice versa).

Importantly, inflammation and blood loss/iron deficiency are not sex-specific and most people have some embodied knowledge of their effects. I subsequently believe that if all children were taught more comprehensive menstrual physiology, this could also help counter the highly problematic PMS gender stereotype. Of course, it might well be that 'Premenstrual Inflammation' (or PMI) becomes the next iteration of the myth of the 'irrational/hysterical/hormonal female' and that the female immune system becomes the next *essence* of femininity used to justify political inequalities. I hope, however, that by revealing the substantial influence of these tropes in biomedical knowledge and practice it might be possible to more easily identify and counter them in the future.

For too long, the 'mystery' surrounding the prevalence of certain symptoms in the female population, especially those that are triggered, worsened or alleviated during reproductive processes (such as the menstrual cycle, pregnancy or the (peri)menopause), has allowed, if not encouraged, the reproduction of biologically reductionist gender myths. Such myths have persisted despite many observable empirical contradictions. Thus, perhaps the main contribution of this research overall is that it helps to shatter the illusion of mystery regarding premenstrual changes and female prevalent symptoms. I hope that by solving this 4,000-year-old riddle, we may one day be able to account for, and attend to, the needs of individual female patients without unintentionally stigmatising 'all women'.

Call to action!

You may feel a little shocked by how little you previously knew about menstrual physiology, the diagnosis of PMS, or the female prevalence of a range of symptoms and conditions. It is not your fault. The omission of crucial information in our school and medical education reflects and reproduces long-standing societal assumptions about femininity. The good news is that we can all do something about these problems right now.

Moving forward in women's health

We need to prevent yet another generation growing up ignorant about our (reproductive) bodies. To my mind this is largely a question of better and more comprehensive education, but each of us, whatever our age, occupation or gender, can do something to help improve this situation.

Research scientists

If working in biomedical research, we must remember that a sub-population prevalence of a certain health condition does not automatically imply a biological (genetic) difference or cause! There is a lot of good quality *biopsychosocial* research out there to support the theory that societal discrimination based on sex, ethnicity, gender, sexuality, socioeconomic status, body type, or any other embodied or political factor, can and will exert a very real impact on an individual's physical and mental health. Instead of shying away from reading critical health research, perhaps we should make doing this a priority? Critical work is not biased or unscientific, it explicitly aims to identify and counter research bias. We do not need to be defensive. It is not our fault that historical and current biomedical education, research and practices are influenced by societal assumptions; nobody is blaming us personally. But it is our responsibility to at least try and counteract such things in our own work.

If working in critical health research, we should seek out and integrate biological, physiological and epidemiological data relevant to our topics. This can only help strengthen our arguments, either by providing supporting evidence or by challenging assumptions within our work. This data is not as difficult to access or comprehend as we may fear! Systematic reviews of the biomedical literature or large-scale epidemiological studies and physiological data from (in)fertility research are a great place to start. The necessary research on women's health issues has already been done in some cases, it just has not filtered through to clinical practice or mainstream biomedical training yet.

If our work involves the 'sex hormones' or some other gendered biological variable, we should be very careful not to unintentionally conflate correlation with causation. Other psychosocial and (non-sex-specific) biological variables may provide a more compelling causal theory. This is relevant to all of us working on perinatal, perimenopausal, women's sports and female-prevalent health topics. Working with an immunologist, or measuring iron stores, inflammatory markers or other (less stereotypically female) hormone levels (serotonin relaxin/cortisol, and so on) before implicating 'oestrogens' or 'progestogens' is always a good idea!

We all need to stick to the available data when conducting research on female-prevalent symptoms or conditions. If a (systematic) review of the literature finds no correlation or causal link between a variable and an outcome, then there likely is none. We should look for an alternative variable rather than trying to prove the data wrong. While it may be tempting to automatically dismiss the validity of other people's work if it challenges our own, we should take a proper look and disprove it using evidence if it is flawed.

Crucially, we need to be especially aware of the use of (unacknowledged) metaphors, as these may end up limiting our ability to verbalise or conceptualise the available data. We should look out for 'hormonal' and 'normal curve/spectrum' analogies in women's health research, in particular.

We also need to remember that the female reproductive body is not only 'for' having children, but also to terminate potentially dangerous or otherwise unviable pregnancies (hence the need to understand sex differences in immune system responses). We should be aware of such pro-natalist assumptions in our training and research activities. Especially since improved understanding the interaction between the immune system and the menstrual cycle could provide novel treatments and cures for a wide range of (female-prevalent) health conditions.

Finally, we need to categorically separate the cyclic triggering or worsening of underlying conditions (medical problems) from the inflammatory changes associated with the menstrual cycle (healthy physiology). More biomedical research is needed on these underlying conditions (especially menstrual health conditions such as endometriosis, adenomyosis, Polycystic Ovary Syndrome, fibroids and heavy menstrual bleeding), but it is simply better *education* that is needed regarding healthy menstrual physiological changes. PMDD should be categorised as another underlying condition, akin to cyclic asthma, catamenial epilepsy and menstrual migraine.

Clinicians and healthcare professionals

We should already be somewhat aware of the problem of unconscious bias when it comes to interactions with patients/clients. When dealing with female-prevalent symptoms and conditions, especially if a patient is Black or of another racialised ethnicity, we need to ensure that we do not (even unintentionally) dismiss or minimise that person's experiences. We should never diminish another person's account of pain. Yes, pain is subjective, but that does not mean that people describing pain, especially if in relation to their reproductive body, are lying or exaggerating for effect. It is probably best to assume that all patients are reliable narrators unless we have a specific and evidence-based reason to doubt their account.[13]

Female-prevalent pain is not 'natural' or 'mysterious', it can and should be explained in the same way as other inflammatory conditions or male experiences of pain. The same goes for female patient descriptions of emotional pain and distress. Rather than automatically blaming the reproductive body and psychologising or minimising patient experiences, we could ask people about what is going on in their lives and/or examine the part of the body they say is in pain, and then do our best to help alleviate their distress. Many of us may feel that we already do this, but the evidence begs to differ.

Someone experiencing severe cyclical mood changes, especially if suicidal, has not just got 'severe PMS'. This comparison is akin to attributing higher male suicide rates to something like 'hanger' (anger/irritability due to hunger). Severe emotional distress stems from distressing experiences, in all humans. Additional factors such as menstrual shame, pain or inflammation (even hanger!) may contribute to distress, but they are unlikely to be the main or only cause. The available evidence suggests that underlying emotional distress/mental health conditions are exacerbated, rather than caused, by cyclic inflammation and blood loss.

If symptoms appear to have a cyclical triggering or worsening, we should ask the patient to track their health over at least two or three cycles before providing a definitive diagnosis. If short appointment times are preventing good practice in this regard, we may need to take collective action (with our colleagues and patients) against such policies.

Psychosocial factors in ill-health are very real and very well-evidenced. Treating our patients as whole human beings, subject to non-biological stressors and risk factors, can only help us to treat them better. Most GPs understand this very well but may feel unable to do much on the psychosocial front due to a lack of resources (time, money, influence). Again, it is really worth fighting together to change these policies and practices to avoid inadequate, stigmatising and ineffective care.

If involved in the development of good practice guidelines, we must remember that as clinicians, we mainly see those with underlying health issues, not the vast majority of people who menstruate without experiencing problematic symptoms. It is not helpful to overstate the prevalence of menstrual health issues in the general population, even if this intuitively feels like the 'right thing to do' to attract more funding or public attention. By exaggerating debility in the female population, we reinforce dangerous and discriminatory beliefs about the 'inherent inferiority' of women in society.

It might be a good idea to approach female patients in the same way that we would approach a man. Perhaps even a specific man? Someone like Dwayne 'The Rock' Johnson? Imagine if The Rock came to you with low (but not technically anaemic) iron levels, fatigue, joint and muscle pain, loss of concentration, and mood changes … and explained how he loses around 40ml of blood every month due to his stunt work, which he hopes will continue for at least another decade. After ruling out anything more serious, I think most of us would readily prescribe iron supplementation, maybe even an intravenous iron transfusion? We would probably also discuss anti-inflammatory pain management options, especially if The Rock described how his symptoms were affecting his quality of life. Given that we need to stop normalising and failing to treat iron deficiency and pain in women and those who menstruate, it could be time to give The Rock method a try? (Please let me know how it goes!)

Wider society

We should always try to speak up when someone implies, jokes about or states that a large population's lived experiences, bodies, decision-making or behaviours are 'natural', 'inherent', 'pathological', 'mysterious', 'exaggerated', 'unreal', 'irrational', 'invented', 'imagined', 'hormonal' or 'hysterical'. These are dangerous political tropes, not facts. Do not underestimate the power of language (especially unacknowledged metaphors) in creating and maintaining discriminatory beliefs and practices.

The reduction and mystification of healthy menstrual physiology in school and medical education has many negative implications for individuals and society as a whole. The really annoying thing is that this is not even difficult science. The cardinal signs of inflammation are well established and clearly exemplified by common premenstrual changes. It is also easy, once we have been taught it, to identify and manage what is happening in our bodies once we know about the purpose and function of periods. We could be taught to recognise an underlying health condition as children, but instead often have to wait over a decade for a diagnosis. This is just not good enough. School and biomedical textbooks need to include more comprehensive menstrual physiology, now!

In fact, I believe that reproductive/menstrual health literacy ought to be a human right. How can we make informed decisions about our health and life choices when we are not taught about the *purpose* of menstruation? If we do not know why humans have periods, and only know them as painful and disruptive experiences, then menstrual taboos and associated discriminatory practices will persist forever. Similarly, if we are not taught about the health risks involved in pregnancy and childbirth, we will continue to make life-changing decisions, without all the necessary information to enable full consent. If we are not taught about the relatively low rate of conception in humans, we will continue to experience great distress if we struggle to conceive. If we are not taught about the high rates of spontaneous abortion in humans – and label them 'miscarriages' – we will continue to unfairly blame the female parent/body for something that is protecting us from harm. If we are not taught about the inflammatory processes involved in the menstrual cycle, we will continue to be mystified by cyclical and female-prevalent symptoms. We will remain mystified by problematic periods, miscarriages, perinatal health conditions and menopausal transitions. We will remain convinced that the female body is (only) 'for' having children, rather than a potential site of conception, contraception and termination – and this belief will be used to justify discrimination against women – whether we want to have children or not.

Box 8.1: Moving forward in women's health: you!

Please share what you have learnt here with your friends, families and other social networks; ask teachers, academics and clinicians to read up on it; share and cite this book and its referenced works; and ask the publishers of textbooks to consider including healthy menstrual physiology (beyond hormones) in their next editions. Together we could help improve the health and wellbeing of half the global human population now and far into the future.

The reduction of menstrual physiology in (medical) education

I reviewed the menstrual cycle content of the most popular school and medical textbooks used in the UK higher education system (King, 2024). The following table is a summary of my findings. Note that brackets denote only a very brief mention of a relevant topic, or a combined rather than separate diagram.

Title	A	B	C	D	E	F	G	H	I	J
1. GCSE Biology AQA (CGP, 2021)	✓	(✓)	✗	✗	✗	✗	✗	✗	✗	✗
2. GCSE Edexcel Biology (CGP, 2017)	✓	(✓)	✗	✗	✗	✗	✗	✗	✗	✗
3. Berne & Levy Physiology, 7th edn (Koeppen and Stanton, 2017)	✓	(✓)	✗	(✓)	(✓)	(✓)	✗	✗	✗	✗
4. Medical Physiology, 3rd edn (Boron and Bouldaep, 2017)	✓	✓	✗	✗	✗	(✓)	✗	(✓)	✗	✗
5. BRS Physiology, 7th edn (Constanzo, 2018a)	✓	✗	✗	✗	✗	✗	✗	(✓)	✗	✗
6. Physiology, 6th edn (Constanzo, 2018b)	✓	✗	✗	✗	✗	✗	✗	(✓)	✗	✗
7. Ganong's Review of Medical Physiology, 7th edn (Barrett et al, 2019)	✓	✓	✗	✗	✗	(✓)	(✓)	(✓)	✗	(✓)
8. Guyton and Hall: Textbook of Medical Physiology, 14th edn (Hall and Hall, 2021)	✓	✓	✗	✗	✗	(✓)	✗	✗	✗	✗
9. Endocrine and Reproductive Physiology, 5th edn (White et al, 2018)	✓	✓	✗	(✓)	✗	(✓)	✗	✗	✗	(✓)
10. Human Reproduction at a Glance, 4th edn (Heffner and Schust, 2014)	✓	(✓)	✗	✗	✗	✗	✗	✗	✗	✗
11. Human Reproductive Biology, 4th edn (Jones and Lopez, 2013)	✓	(✓)	✗	✗	✓	✗	(✓)	(✓)	(✓)	(✓)
12. Knobil and Neill's Physiology of Reproduction, 4th edn (Plant and Zeleznik, 2015)	✓	✓	✗	✓	✗	✗	✗	(✓)	✓	✗
13. Oxford Textbook of Obstetrics and Gynaecology (Whitaker et al, 2020)	✓	(✓)	✗	(✓)	✓	✓	✗	✗	(✓)	(✓)
14. Oxford Handbook of General Practice (Simon et al, 2014)	✓	✗	✗	✗	✓	(✓)	✓	✗	(✓)	✓
15. Oxford Handbook of Obstetrics and Gynaecology (Collins et al, 2013)	✓	(✓)	✗	✗	✓	(✓)	✗	✗	(✓)	✓
16. Routledge International Handbook of Women's Sexual and Reproductive Health (Ussher et al, 2019)	✓	✗	✗	✗	✓	✓	✗	(✓)	✗	✓

Notes: A: diagram showing hormonal level changes associated with the menstrual cycle; B: diagram showing uterine changes associated with the menstrual cycle; C: theorised abortifacient purpose of menstruation; D: inflammatory nature of cyclical physiological events; E: pain; F: blood loss; G: swelling/water retention; H: temperature increase; I: iron-deficiency anaemia; J: menstrual health issues – Premenstrual Syndrome, endometriosis, heavy bleeding, migraine, and so on.

Participant background survey

This short survey is part of the research project 'A comparison of professional and patient descriptions of Premenstrual Syndrome (PMS)'. Answering these questions will help to provide some context to what is said in the interviews. This data will be made anonymous and generalised so nobody will be able to identify who you are. You also do not have to answer any of these questions. Personal information is only requested because it may have an influence upon the way in which you experience or describe PMS. Ethical Clearance Reference Number: MRSP-19/20-14792.

1. **Please indicate your sex:** Female/Intersex/Male/Prefer not to say.
2. **Please indicate your gender identity:** Woman/Non-binary (or Other)/Man/Prefer not to say.
3. **Please select the age group to which you belong**: Under 18/ 18–24/25–34/35–44/45–54/55–64/65+/Prefer not to say.
4. **Do you currently have children under the age of 18 living in your household?** Y/N/Prefer not to say.
5. **If so, how many?** 1/2/3/4 or more/Prefer not to say.
6. **What best describes your marital status?** Single, not married, no partner/Single, not married, partner living elsewhere/Living with partner/Married/Separated/Divorced/Widowed/Prefer not to say.
7. **What best describes your sexual orientation?** Straight/Gay/ Lesbian/Bisexual/Other/Prefer not to say.
8. **What best describes your employment status?** Full-time parent/ Employed – full-time/Employed – part-time/Student/Not employed – looking for work/Not employed – not looking for work/Retired/Prefer not to say.
9. **What best describes your level of education?** Primary school only/ Some secondary school/Secondary school (up to GCSEs)/Sixth form or college (A levels, NVQs)/Professional qualification (equivalent to degree level)/University – undergraduate degree/University – postgraduate degree/University – MD (Medical Degree)/Prefer not to say.
10. **If you have an academic or medical qualification(s), please indicate the subject(s):**
11. **In which country do you live?** [Self-defined]/Prefer not to say.
12. **What is your ethnicity?** [Self-defined]/Prefer not to say.
13. **Were you brought up within a religious household?** Yes/No/ Prefer not to say.
14. **If so, what religion?** [Self-defined]/Prefer not to say.

15. **Are you currently affiliated with any religion?** Yes/No/Prefer not to say.
16. **If so, what religion?** [Self-defined]/Prefer not to say.
17. **What is your approximate annual household income?** Under £20,000/£20K–£29K/£30K–£39K/£40K–£49K/£50K–£59K/£60K–£69K/£70K–£79K/£80K or more/Prefer not to say.

Interview question lists

Expert interview schedule

PMS

E1. How did you come to be interested in premenstrual syndrome (PMS)?

E2. How would you describe 'PMS' to someone who has never heard of it?

E3. Do/did you/any close family members identify as someone who experiences PMS?

E4. How did you first come to know about PMS?

E5. How common is PMS?

E6. What is your understanding of *why* premenstrual symptoms occur?

E7. In your opinion, what is the best way to manage PMS?

E8. Are you aware of any societal stereotype of someone with PMS? If so, can you describe it?

Symptoms

E9. In your understanding, roughly how many premenstrual symptoms are there?

E10. In your understanding, what are the most common premenstrual symptoms? Could you perhaps list a top ten?

E11. What is your understanding about the difference(s) between PMS and PMDD?

E12. Would you consider period pain as a premenstrual symptom? Why?

E13. In your opinion what does the premenstrual symptom 'bloating' specifically refer to?

E14. Many chronic health conditions get worse at certain times in the menstrual cycle. Would you count the expression of these as premenstrual symptoms? Why?

E15. Are there any positive menstrual changes? If so, what are they?

E16. Men can also experience nearly all of the same symptoms described as being associated with PMS, just without any cyclical pattern. Do the same symptoms therefore have different biological mechanisms, depending on the patient's sex?

Diagnostic and therapeutic controversies

E17. PMS is considered by some to be a controversial diagnosis – what is your understanding of why this might be?

E18. The latest (ISPMD consensus-based) guidelines on PMS state that 'any' symptoms count, so long as they occur in the luteal phase, resolve shortly after menstruation begins, and are severe enough to affect daily life. How do you feel about this particular definition?

E19. Such guidelines on PMS also promote the use of symptom tracking tools in order to assist formal diagnosis. However, the most popular tools are based on the specific symptoms associated with the DSM diagnostic criteria for PMDD. What do you think about this?

E20. The guidelines categorise PMDD as a core premenstrual disorder alongside PMS rather than as a mental health disorder that is triggered or worsened at certain points in the menstrual cycle. What do you think about this?

E21. Clinical guidelines on PMS do not usually include information about the role of non-biological or external life experiences as contributing factors in menstrual cycle-related health, for example, 'psycho-social' factors. What do you think about that?

E22. PMDD is categorised as a mental health disorder, and yet its specific diagnostic criteria include several normal physical menstrual changes/symptoms – what do you think about that?

E23. What do you think about the use of diuretics (Spironolactone) in the treatment of PMS?

E24. What do you think about surgical interventions in the treatment of PMS/PMDD?

Evaluation

E25. [Optional and eventually discarded] I think it is possible to better integrate the various clinical, academic and patient discourses – to inform an evidence-based and standardised list of cyclical symptoms. How do you rate my chances?

E26. How do you feel about this interview? Do you have any questions or comments you would like to add?

Patient interview schedule

Periods

P1. Growing up, how did your family talk about periods?

P2. What was your first period like?

P3. Do you feel different before, during or after your period?

P4. Do you do anything special, or refrain from doing anything, around your period?

P5. Does your period affect you at home, work or socially?

P6. How would you describe periods to a child?

P7.   What is your understanding of *why* periods occur?

P8.   Do periods have any religious, spiritual or any other special or symbolic significance for you?

P9.   Overall, how do you feel about periods and the fact that you get them for about 40 years?

P10. If you could wave a magic wand to get rid of your periods, would you?

PMS

P11. Do you identify as someone who gets PMS?

P12. How did you first come to know about PMS?

P13. How would you describe PMS to someone who had never heard of it?

P14. How common is PMS do you think?

P15. What is your understanding of why premenstrual symptoms occur?

P16. How do you manage your symptoms?

P17. Have you ever consulted a doctor about your experiences? If so, how did that go?

P18. Do you think doctors have enough knowledge/training on menstrual cycle-related symptoms?

P19. Is there a stereotype of a person with PMS?

P20. Have you ever heard of PMDD, Premenstrual Dysphoric Disorder? If so, what is your understanding about the difference between PMS and PMDD?

Symptoms

P21. Do you track your menstrual cycle-related symptoms?

P22. In your own understanding, roughly how many premenstrual symptoms are there?

P23. In your understanding, what are the most common premenstrual symptoms? Could you perhaps list a top ten?

P24. Would you consider period pain as a premenstrual symptom? Why?

P25. What does the term 'bloating' mean to you?

P26. Do you have any other health conditions that get worse at certain times in the menstrual cycle? If so, would you count these as premenstrual symptoms?

P27. Which symptoms do you experience nearly every cycle?

P28. Have your typical symptoms changed over time?

P29. Are you aware of PMS being a controversial diagnosis? [Follow up] Have you ever met someone who didn't believe you were really experiencing these symptoms?

P30. Have you ever experienced any positive menstrual changes?

Evaluation

P31. How do you feel about this conversation? Has it made you feel, or think any differently than you did before?

Transcription notation

The transcription notation used in this study was adapted from that first proposed by Gail Jefferson in her 'Glossary of transcript symbols with an introduction' (Jefferson, 2004). Adapted symbols are highlighted in bold.

The last four listed conventions relating to speed and intonation were not used (due to time constraints and infrequent/unremarkable usage).

Transcription notation

(.)	A full stop inside brackets denotes a notable pause but of less than one second in length.
(pause)	'Pause' written inside brackets denotes a pause between one and three seconds in length.
(long pause)	'Long pause' written inside brackets denotes a pause over three seconds in length.
=	The equal sign denotes latched speech, no gap between words or speakers.
:	Colons denote elongated speech, a stretched sound.
CAPITALS	Something that was said loudly or even shouted.
(whispering)	Something that was said very quietly or in a purposeful whisper
Underlined	When a word or part of a word is underlined it denotes a raise in volume or emphasis.
(laugh)	When a bracketed 'laugh' appears it means that there was laughter within or around the talk.
(inhale)	Denotes audible intake of breath.
(exhale)	Denotes audible exhalation of breath.
(sigh)	Denotes audible sigh with element of voice.
'yes'	Single quotation marks denote reported speech or thought.
[Square brackets]	denote a point where overlapping speech occurs.
(( ))	Double brackets denote some contextual information where no symbol of representation was available.
( )	Where there is space between brackets denotes that the words spoken here were too unclear to transcribe.
> <	Arrows surrounding talk denote that the pace of the speech has quickened.
< >	Arrows in this direction denote that the pace of the speech has slowed down.
↑	When an upward arrow appears it means there is a rise in intonation.
↓	When a downward arrow appears it means there is a drop in intonation.

Discursive device notation

The 20 discursive devices annotated during this study are those listed by Sally Wiggins (2017). The seven devices that emerged as being of most analytical interest are highlighted in bold font, while those that were of less importance are shaded in grey.

Device name	Description and example function
Pronoun use and footing shifts	Using different pronouns (I, we, you, us, one) can highlight the relationship between the speaker and the account they are providing. Footing shifts refer to the way in which we might speak as the author, animator or principle of the discourse.
Assessments and second assessments	Assessments (evaluations) in interaction are often followed by second assessments; these are typically upgraded if they agree with the first assessment. There is a 'preference structure' for assessments.
Silences, pauses and hesitations	Silences/pauses can indicate trouble in interaction; if there are too many pauses or too long a gap between speakers.
Hedging	Hedging talk often precedes a dis-preferred second assessment (that is, a second assessment that disrupts conversational norms); it can also be seen in accounts, and can function to highlight the delicacy of an issue.
Extreme case formulations (ECF)	A phrase or word that is semantically extreme; that is, invoking the maximal or minimal properties of an object, person or event. Can be used to justify or strengthen an argument, add credibility and manage one's identity.
Minimisation	Treats the object or account as minimal, often using the terms 'just', 'only', 'little', 'bit'. Can be used to downplay the significance or importance of something.
Lists and contrasts	Listing is a regular feature of interaction, and three-part lists add a particular rhetorical strength to an argument. They are often used in political speeches for this reason. Contrast can be setting up an either/or state of affairs, or contrasting the speaker's intentions/desires without alternative 'reality'. In both cases, they can be used to manage accountability and identities.
Affect displays	Displaying affect (that is, an emotive or physical state) in interaction is often organised within the unfolding interaction, for example, immediately preceding or following a particular action in the interaction.
Consensus and corroboration	These are accounts that suggest that many people or everyone agrees with what you are saying (consensus) or that someone else provides an independent witness (corroboration). Both of these are key ways in which people can attend to the factuality of what they are saying and reduce any sense of their own investment in the account.

Device name	Description and example function
Detail versus vagueness	Giving specific details of an event or person versus being vague or unclear can manage investment ('stake') in the account and thus the speaker's entitlement to tell the account or to be asked questions about it. It can also be used to suggest particular observation skills on the part of the speaker (that is, their identity as being accurate and observant).
Disclaimers	These are inserted statements before the main account to try to mitigate the speaker's stance on a particular issue. They make visible a particular interpretation of what they are going to say, then explicitly deny this. These often work alongside category membership-type issues (that is, when a speaker's identity is being explicitly addressed).
Metaphor	Metaphors can be subtle or more striking, and they can frame an account in a particular way, opening up issues of agency and blame, as well as speaker categories and footing.
Narrative structure	Presenting an account in a sequential order and within a particular temporal structure; often highlights things that need to be known first. The plausibility of an account can also be increased by embedding the account in a narrative sequence.
Reported speech (aka active voicing)	Where speakers report the words or thoughts of others as if they were directly spoken; adds authenticity to an account.
Script formulations	This is where an account appears as if it is a regular or frequent occurrence (as if scripted or following a script); can present the account as normal and expected.
Agent subject distinction	Speakers often make relevant their agency within a particular course of events; that is, how they are positioned as active or passive, and their associated responsibility or accountability for these events. This is also related to 'empiricist reporting', where academic articles are written in the third person to remove any sense of research agency or subjectivity.
Emotion categories	Speakers often make reference to their own or other people's emotional states. In discursive research these are analysed in terms of their interactional function, as a discursive accomplishment rather than as indicating an underlying emotional state.
Category entitlements	Using a category to refer to a person or category bound activity (for example, age, gender, job or career, family position); inferences can be made from either categories of persons or activities and who might or might not be expected to engage in such activities.
Modal verbs	Modal verbs are those that infer obligations, abilities or likelihood of something; as such, they can be used to manage responsibility or accountability for one's own or other people's actions.
Stake inoculation	Similar to category entitlements, this is where speakers construct their talk to defend against the claim that they might have a stake in what they are saying (that is, that they might be biased or subjective).

Discourse coding tree

Themes (n=4)

1. Psychologising premenstrual change (Chapter 4).
2. Premenstrual change as simultaneously normal and debilitating (Chapter 5).
3. Femininity as debility (Chapter 6).
4. Lack of/contradictory knowledge about healthy menstrual physiology (Chapter 7).

Axial codes (n=42)

Theme one is comprised of:

1. Descriptions of symptoms/PMS/PMDD psychological causality/ontological claims.
2. Differentiating PMS/PMDD/PME of mental health disorders.
3. Biomedical expert reluctance to self-ID with PMS.
4. Inclusion of physical symptoms in descriptions of PMS.
5. PMS as emotional distress caused by premenstrual changes.
6. Prioritisation of mood symptoms in descriptions of PMS.
7. Relationship between PMS/PMDD.
8. Societal depictions of PMS as stigmatising/mood-based/all in the mind.
9. Suicide as more urgent/serious than other changes.
10. Switching between biomedical and stereotypical definitions of PMS.

Theme two is comprised of:

1. Dysmenorrhea/period pain as separate from PMS.
2. Interdisciplinary disagreement.
3. Internalisation of societal depictions of PMS.
4. Medical justifications for prioritising mood change.
5. Medicalisation as a negative thing.
6. Minimising experiences/laughter/language.
7. Normal curve/spectrum analogies.
8. Patient experiences of disbelief.
9. PMS is not an illness.
10. PMS/PMDD as unique/temporary.
11. Problematic definition of PMDD.

Theme three is comprised of:

1. All women have PMS.
2. Binary sex differences – categorical distinctions made.
3. Exaggerated prevalence/# symptoms/severity.
4. Feminine attributes as problematic – weight/skin/appetite/libido/emotional expression.
5. Gender stereotype of PMS – hysterical/irrational/hypochondriac female.
6. Hysterectomy as a problematic/cure for emotional distress.
7. Menstrual cycle as cause of PMS/PMDD.
8. Periods as a negative/curse/dirty/stressful/shameful.
9. Pure PMS/PMDD.
10. Sex/hormones as cause of symptoms/PMS/PMDD.

Theme four is comprised of:

1. Hormonal causal explanations.
2. Binary sex differences – categorical distinctions made.
3. Differentiating normal changes from pathological changes.
4. Female body as mysterious/unknowable/too complex.
5. Feminists quoting biomedical discourse.
6. Lack of education re: periods/PMS/physiology – GPs, patients, specialists.
7. Lifestyle/dietary options for treatment of PMS.
8. Normal changes as unknown.
9. PMS as contested between disciplines – definition/ownership/medicalisation.

Open codes (n=75)

1. All women have PMS.
2. Binary sex differences are categorical.
3. Blame feminists for disbelief in PMS/PMDD.
4. Blame gynaecology for definitional issues.
5. Blame psychiatry for definitional issues.
6. Variation across reproductive lifetime.
7. Contradictory nature of definitions.
8. Disbelief in physiological basis for symptoms.
9. Disbelief in reality of PMS.
10. Disbelief in severity of symptoms.
11. Contested disciplinary ownership of PMS/PMDD.
12. DSM definition of PMDD as arbitrary.
13. DSM definition of PMDD as medicalising.
14. Exaggerated number of symptoms.

15. Exaggerated prevalence of PMS.
16. Reluctance to self-ID with PMS.
17. External/psychosocial factors as causal in PMS/PMDD.
18. Familial disbelief in experiences.
19. Feminine attributes as problematic – weight/skin/appetite/libido/emotion.
20. Gender norms inform PMS/PMDD.
21. Gender stereotype of PMS – hysterical/irrational/hypochondriac female.
22. Hysterectomy as a (problematic) cure for emotional distress.
23. PMS as biological/physiological.
24. Internalisation of societal depictions of PMS/gender.
25. Lack of clinical training for GPs.
26. Lack of education re: periods/PMS.
27. Lack of research/evidence.
28. Lifestyle/dietary management of PMS.
29. PMS as magical/mysterious/spiritual/unknowable.
30. Media portrayal of PMS stereotypes.
31. PMS diagnosis as difficult.
32. Medical disbelief in experiences.
33. PMS medications/treatment options.
34. Menopause as scary/liberating.
35. Menstrual cycle/hormones as cause of symptoms/PMS/PMDD.
36. Menstruation taboo/secrecy/shame.
37. Misdiagnosis as common.
38. Normal changes as unknown.
39. Common normal changes.
40. Normal curve/spectrum analogies.
41. Other menstrual health issues.
42. Familial disbelief in experiences.
43. Pain as subjective.
44. Period pain as inevitable.
45. PMS as crazy/irrational experience.
46. Period pain as (not) PMS.
47. Periods as negative/the curse/painful/stressful/shameful.
48. Personal responsibility to manage premenstrual experiences/health.
49. Physical changes as less debilitating.
50. Physical changes as not what patients seek help for.
51. PMDD as more severe PMS.
52. Most common PMDD symptoms.
53. PMS as any and all changes.
54. PMS as contested between disciplines.
55. PMS as normal.
56. Most common PMS symptoms.

57. PMS/normal changes as 'less severe' form of PMDD.
58. Positive premenstrual changes.
59. Premenstrual exacerbation – migraine/asthma/epilepsy/fibroids/anaemia.
60. The prioritisation of mood symptoms in descriptions of PMS.
61. Pure or core PMS/PMDD.
62. RCOG definition of PMS as good/inclusive.
63. RCOG definition of PMS as problematic/medicalising.
64. Relationship between PMS/PMDD.
65. Sensitivity to hormones/allergy hypothesis.
66. Severe experiences as PMS.
67. Sex/hormones as cause of emotion.
68. Some patients are excluded from PMS/PMDD definitions.
69. Suicide/psychosis/extreme mood change as hormonal in origin.
70. The temporary nature of premenstrual changes.
71. Most common/effective treatment types.
72. Vagueness of PMS definition as problematic.
73. Individual variation in experiences/over time.
74. Menstruation as dirty/toxic.
75. Menstruation as 'prepping for pregnancy'.

The influence of three key gender myths on the participant group discourses

Biomedical PMS experts

Biomedical PMS experts (n=13)

---

1. **Femininity as debility**
    • Debilitating symptoms positioned as simply 'more severe' versions of healthy cyclical changes (normal curve analogy).
    • Inclusion of typically mild physical changes in definitions of PMS and PMDD.
    • Symptoms are attributed to the female sex hormones.
    • Number and prevalence of debilitating symptoms is exaggerated.
    • Positioning of hysterectomy as 'cure' for severely debilitating symptoms.

2. **All in her mind**
    • Mood changes prioritised over physical changes.
    • PMDD positioned as 'severe PMS' (but cyclical asthma/epilepsy are not).
    • Three pain symptoms are minimised, including 'period pain'.
    • Severe physical cyclical symptoms are categorised as inherently 'less debilitating' and something 'other' than PMS.
    • Positioning of PMS (as opposed to PMDD) as a mental health condition.
    • Psychiatry's clinical ownership of PMS (as well as PMDD).

3. **The mysterious female (reproductive) body**
    • Emotional distress is attributed to the female (hormonal) body, not life circumstances.
    • The reduction of the menstrual cycle to (female sex) hormonal fluctuations, only, omitting most of the physiological processes involved.
    • Contradictory epidemiological data regarding the assumed causal role of the female sex hormones positioned as mysterious rather than indicative of alternative mechanism(s).
    • Dismissal of 'feminist' critical literature regarding psychosocial factors in PMS.
    • Endorsement of 'no symptoms listed' in formal PMS diagnostic guidelines.

Critical PMS experts ('quoted' biomedical discourses are indicated by square brackets)

Critical PMS experts (n=3)

---

1. Femininity as debility
- Debilitating symptoms positioned as simply 'more severe' versions of healthy cyclical changes (normal curve analogy).
- Endorsement of the inclusion of typically mild physical changes in definitions of PMS and PMDD by two of the group.
- [Symptoms are attributed to the female sex hormones.]
- [Number of debilitating symptoms exaggerated by one of the group.]

2. All in her mind
- Mood changes prioritised over physical changes.
- [PMDD positioned as 'severe PMS' by two of the group.]
- Three pain symptoms are minimised, including 'period pain'.
- [Severe physical cyclical symptoms are categorised as inherently 'less debilitating' and something 'other' than PMS.]
- Psychology's academic ownership of critical PMS research.

3. The mysterious female (reproductive) body
- [The reduction of the menstrual cycle to (female sex) hormonal fluctuations, only, omitting most of the physiological processes involved.]
- Endorsement of 'no symptoms listed' in formal PMS diagnostic guidelines by two of the group.

PMS patients

PMS patients (n=12)

---

1. Femininity as debility
- Debilitating symptoms positioned as simply 'more severe' versions of healthy cyclical changes (normal curve analogy).
- Changes associated with an idealised femininity (especially body image) prioritised over others.
- Symptoms are attributed to the female sex hormones.
- All changes described as PMS and so population prevalence is exaggerated (although half the group stated that it is 'not an illness').
- Positioning of menstruation as 'toxic'.

2. All in her mind
- PMDD positioned as 'severe PMS' by the seven patients who had heard of PMDD.
- Two pain symptoms are minimised (headache and muscle/joint pain).

3. The mysterious female (reproductive) body
- Explicit lack of knowledge about menstrual physiology.
- Positioning of premenstrual changes as 'crazy' or 'weird'.
- The reduction of the menstrual cycle to (female sex) hormonal fluctuations.

Notes

Introduction

1. Cordage (1684).
2. Putnam Jacobi (1876).
3. Horney (1967).
4. de Beauvoir (2010).
5. Martin (1987).
6. Walker (1997).
7. Laws et al (1985); Laws (1990).
8. Caplan (1995).
9. Figert (1996).
10. Chrisler and Caplan (2002); Chrisler and Gorman (2015).
11. Ussher (2005, 2011).
12. Ussher and Perz (2013a, 2020a, 2020b).
13. DeLuca (2017).
14. https://beta.ukdataservice.ac.uk/datacatalogue/studies/study?id=855486
15. Gunter (2024, pp 10, 116).
16. King (2024).
17. Bobel (2010); Weiss-Wolf (2017).
18. De Benedictis (2023, pp 886–887).
19. Tax Policy Associates (2022).
20. Bobel (2019, pp 282–285).
21. King (2021, 2023).
22. King (2021, 2023).
23. *BBC News Online* (2020); Khan (2023).
24. Miller (2022).
25. Taylor et al (2018); As-Sanie et al (2019); Westwood et al (2023).
26. Weisse et al (2001); Wandner et al (2012); Williams et al (2015); Palacios-Ceña et al (2017).
27. Mukwende et al (2020).
28. *BBC Newsround* (2020).
29. Clark et al (2023).
30. www.menstrual-matters.com
31. King (2020).
32. https://beta.ukdataservice.ac.uk/datacatalogue/studies/study?id=855486

Chapter 1

1. King (2024).
2. Martin (1987).
3. CGP (2017, 2021).
4. CGP (2017, 2021).
5. CGP (2017, 2021).
6. King (2024).
7. King (2024).
8. The word 'abortion' is the proper term used to describe the expulsion of the contents of the womb and has been for centuries. Miscarriages were known as 'spontaneous abortions' right up until the beginning of the 20th century. Abortions initiated by medications or surgery are more properly described as 'medical' or 'surgical' abortions.

9   Emera et al (2012).

10 When dogs are on heat, this is not the same thing as a period. In their case, they secrete a bloody fluid from the vaginal wall (not the womb) during ovulation to communicate to other dogs that they are fertile. In stark contrast, humans conceal ovulation and bleed from the womb two weeks later. No more sexist comparisons between menstruating women and bitches on heat, please!

11 Critchley et al (2020, p 629).

12 Emera et al (2012); Bellofiore and Evans (2019).

13 Emera et al (2012).

14 Emera et al (2012).

15 Emera et al (2012).

16 A quick note on the word 'theory'. In scientific terms, the word refers to an idea that is well supported by the available evidence. Popular conceptions of 'theory' often wrongly mistake it for a 'hypothesis' – a preliminary idea still to be tested, or one that currently lacks substantial supporting evidence.

17 Brosens et al (2022).

18 Regan and Rai (2000, p 840).

19 Jarvis (2016, p 9).

20 WHO (2023).

21 King (2024, pp 31–32).

22 Tan et al (2017).

23 Fraser et al (2001).

24 Salamonsen (2021). In fact, menstrual fluid-derived stem cells helped save the lives of some critically ill patients during the COVID-19 pandemic (Xu et al, 2021).

25 WHO (2023).

26 Johnston-Robledo and Chrisler (2013).

27 King (2024).

28 Here are the other two previous hypotheses for those keen to know: one is that menstruation helps to get rid of pathogens brought into the womb by sperm during heterosexual sex. The problems identified with this idea were that periods can occur weeks after sex, and that sperm-borne pathogens are not unique to menstruating species. I would additionally argue that the cumulative blood loss associated with periods likely weakens our immune system, which seems counterintuitive if they evolved to eliminate pathogens. The remaining hypothesis claims that having regular periods is less costly than maintaining a thickened womb lining over time. The main problem with this idea is that no mammals maintain a thickened womb lining over time! Most experience the decidualisation/thickening process only in response to an embryo attaching to the womb lining. I would also argue that ovulation, SD and menstruation *are* very costly when it comes to energy expenditure. After all, the cycle is highly inflammatory, painful and involves significant blood loss (approximately 20 litres or 44 pints) over the average 40 years. Considering that an average human body contains only five litres or 11 pints of blood, this is a big deal!

29 Emera et al (2012).

30 WHO (2023).

31 Robillard et al (2019).

32 Pinho and Gaunt (2024).

33 Bull et al (2019).

34 Robillard et al (2002).

35 Simmons and Jennings (2020, pp 69–70).

36 The categorisation of the so-called 'sex' hormones as either male or female is misleading. All humans have both types of hormones, the levels of which only differ by *average*

circulating levels and fluctuate continuously, throughout the day, with age, in different parts of the body, in response to external stimuli, and in the case of females, also in relation to the menstrual cycle during our reproductive years. Yet, this information runs contrary to popular and historical scientific opinion (Oudshoorn, 2003, pp 22–37). In fact, the highest concentration of oestrone (three times the level typically found in circulation at the peak of ovulation) is found in the male testes (Hess et al, 1997, p 509). More representative names for the sex hormones might be the 'fertility' or 'reproductive' hormones, given their crucial role in the development of secondary sexual characteristics and maintenance of male and female reproductive health.

[37] Rubinow and Schmidt (2006); RCOG (2016); Zendehdel and Elyasi (2018).

[38] Rubinow et al (1988); Rubinow and Schmidt (1995, 2006).

[39] RCOG (2016, p 80).

[40] Segebladh et al (2009).

[41] Schaffir et al (2016).

[42] Hess et al (1997); King and Critchley (2010); Maybin and Critchley (2015).

[43] Espey (1980).

[44] Casimiri and Psychoyos (1981).

[45] Finn (1986).

[46] Abrams and Miller (2011).

[47] Barabás et al (2020).

[48] Ojeda-Ojeda et al (2013); Schmidt et al (2014); Shorakae et al (2018).

[49] Maybin et al (2011); Maybin and Critchley (2015); Whitaker et al (2020).

[50] Rier and Yeaman (2008); Christodoulakos et al (2009); Farland et al (2017).

[51] Modugno et al (2005); Yu et al (2009).

[52] Gao et al (2021).

[53] Tang and Wang (2018, p 295).

[54] Shattuck and Muehlenbein (2015); Critchley and Garfinkel (2017); Harrison (2017).

[55] Graziottin and Serafini (2016).

[56] Bellei et al (2020).

[57] Rana and Musto (2018).

[58] Majd et al (2020).

[59] Renna et al (2018).

[60] Bertone-Johnson et al (2014); Bertone-Johnson (2016); Gold et al (2016).

[61] Gold et al (2016, p 866).

[62] RCOG (2016).

[63] Collao et al (2020).

[64] Lopresti (2017).

[65] Stach et al (2021).

[66] Makabe et al (2017).

[67] Dionisie et al (2021).

[68] Mohammadi et al (2022).

[69] Marjoribanks et al (2015); Behboudi-Gandevani et al (2018); Hafiz et al (2018); Potter et al (2021). Note: ibuprofen or Omega 3 supplements both work really well in terms of reducing menstrual blood loss and period pain. But, if you try this approach and it does not work for you, please seek medical advice as you may have an underlying health issue, such as adenomyosis, endometriosis, fibroids or heavy menstrual bleeding.

[70] Marván and Escobedo (1999); Ussher (2004); Kleinstäuber et al (2012, 2016); Smorgick et al (2013); Balik et al (2014); van Iersel et al (2016).

[71] Klyne et al (2021).

[72] Hancock et al (2015).

[73] Percy et al (2017).

74 NICE (2023). Mathematical, as opposed to physiological/clinical calculations of 'normal' iron levels are currently:
  • In men aged over 15 years – Hb below 130 g/L.
  • In non-pregnant women aged over 15 years – Hb below 120 g/L.
  • In pregnant women – Hb below 110 g/L throughout pregnancy.
  • Postpartum (after giving birth) – Hb below 100 g/L.
75 Dugan et al (2021).
76 Roberts and Jones (2023).
77 Dugan et al (2021).
78 Dugan et al (2021); Roberts and Jones (2023).
79 Cappellini et al (2020).
80 Sinha et al (2013); Angeli et al (2016).
81 Chocano-Bedoya et al (2013); Sinha et al (2013); Zeitoun et al (2021). The anonymous data I have collected (from over 1,500 people) via the 'symptom checker' app on the Menstrual Matters website also suggest a relationship between low iron levels and cyclical symptoms of all types.
82 King (2024).
83 Mirin (2021).
84 As-Sanie et al (2019).
85 Hoffmann and Tarzian (2001); Weisse et al (2001); Wandner et al (2012); Orhan et al (2018).
86 Westwood et al (2023).
87 Sharma et al (2022).
88 Taylor (2006); Palacios-Ceña et al (2017); Westwood et al (2023).
89 Ussher (2005).
90 Pinho and Gaunt (2024).
91 Brosens et al (2022).

Chapter 2

1 Veith (1965); Micale (2019).
2 Gilman et al (1993); Devereux (2014).
3 Laws et al (1985).
4 Quirke (2002, ll. 1–29).
5 Hippocrates of Cos (2018).
6 Hippocrates of Cos (2018, pp 32–33).
7 Hippocrates of Cos (2018, pp 122–123).
8 Quirke (2002); Hippocrates of Cos (2018, p 15).
9 Ussher (1989); King (1998).
10 King (1993, 1998).
11 Veith (1965, p 122). Tellingly, the idea that Hippocratic 'hysteria' referred to modern definitions of excessive emotion or irrational behaviour (rather than physical symptoms only) is also reproduced in scholarly publications spanning a range of academic/clinical disciplines. For example, medical history (Micale, 2019), critical health psychology (Tasca et al, 2012), psychiatry (Brulin-Solignac et al, 2021), psychoanalysis (Grose, 2016), gynaecology (O'Brien and Ismail, 2007) and neurology (Trimble and Reynolds, 2016).
12 Gilman et al (1993, p 143).
13 Micale (2019, p 22).
14 Veith (1965, p 141).
15 Latham (1848).

[16] Jules Falret, a physician treating 'hysterics' at the infamous Salpêtrière hospital, in 1866, as cited in Veith (1965, p 211).

[17] Freud and Breuer (1895).

[18] Veith (1965, p 265).

[19] Micale (2019, p 29).

[20] Veith (1965, p 174).

[21] Ávila and Terra (2012).

[22] Letson and Dancey (1996); Hoffmann and Tarzian (2001); Asbring and Närvänen (2002); Palacios-Ceña et al (2017).

[23] King (1998).

[24] Cordage (1684, p 69).

[25] Willis (1667, cited in Cordage, 1684, p 69).

[26] It is worth noting that Simone de Beauvoir previously outlined much the same argument in *The Second Sex*, published in 1949 (de Beauvoir, 2010).

[27] Gilman et al (1993); King (1998); Devereux (2014).

[28] Lloyd (1984); Pateman (1988); Fraisse (1994).

[29] Greer (1999); Ehrenreich and English (2011). Since 1981, the term *hysteria* has also been 'reclaimed' by several literary scholars, authors and filmmakers using 'hysterical narrative' to contend that 19th-century hysterics were proto-feminists, expressing resistance to patriarchal gender norms through their bodies. This metaphorical interpretation of the term hysteria falls beyond the scope of my physiological argument, but a useful summary of such work (and its critics) is provided by Devereux (2014).

[30] Martin (1987); Federici (2004).

[31] Duby and Perrot (1993).

[32] Lloyd (1984).

[33] Lloyd (1984); Fricker and Hornsby (2001).

[34] Lloyd (1984).

[35] Descartes (1637).

[36] Federici (2004, p 8).

[37] King (2020).

[38] Myers (2014).

[39] Laws et al (1985).

[40] Stepan (1986).

[41] Saguy et al (2021); Roth et al (2023).

[42] Stepan (1986, p 270).

[43] Friedan (1963, p 127).

[44] Williams et al (2003).

[45] Laws et al (1985); Ussher (2011).

[46] Howard and Howard (2022).

[47] Oudshoorn (2003, p 55).

[48] Frank (1929, p 1). In her most recent book on the history of women's health and medicine, Helen King (2024, p 292) adds more context to Frank's choice of Latin subtitle. The phrase was first used by eminent British gynaecologist, William Blair Bell, during a public lecture in 1913. Blair Bell was himself responding to an earlier adage attributed to Jan Baptist van Helmont; *propter solum uterum mulier est quod est*, 'it is because of the womb alone that woman is what she is', which was most likely Helmont's version of 4th-century BCE Hippocratic texts that positioned the womb was 'the origin of all diseases of women'. This discursive history wonderfully illustrates the millennia-old medical tendency to blame biological markers of 'femininity' for female-prevalent symptoms, rather than looking for non-sex-specific physiological causes.

[49] Frank (1931).

[50] Frank (1931, p 1054).

[51] O'Brien and Ismail (2007).

[52] Veith (1965); Laws et al (1985); Rodin (1992).

[53] Stepan (1986, p 264).

[54] Greene and Dalton (1953).

[55] Dalton (1964, pp 7–15).

[56] King (2020).

[57] Dalton (1969, pp 129–132).

[58] O'Brien and Ismail (2007).

[59] O'Brien and Ismail (2007).

[60] Gao et al (2021, p 4).

[61] Boorse (1987); Chrisler and Levy (1990); Chrisler and Caplan (2002).

[62] Harry and Balcer (1987).

[63] APA (1987).

[64] King (2020).

[65] RCOG (2016, p 80; emphasis added).

[66] Dennerstein et al (2009, 2011); Mallia (2015).

[67] RCOG (2016, p 81).

[68] We see exactly the same pattern in clinical research and popular beliefs regarding (peri)
natal and (peri)menopausal mood disorders – where, again, there is insufficient evidence
to position either of the female sex hormones as a direct causal factor (in fact, oestrogen
appears to be a protective factor against depression), but plenty of evidence to show
how non-sex specific factors contribute to an individual's risk of illness. For instance,
previous experiences of mood disorders/emotional distress/violent trauma, experiences
of racism/xenophobia/sexism, lack of spousal or social support, inflammation, iron-
deficiency anaemia, and other underlying chronic health issues (Avis et al, 2018; Cannon
and Nasrallah, 2019; Payne and Maguire, 2019; Wassef et al, 2019). Again, symptom
correlation with changes in reproductive hormone levels does not in itself prove causation,
and yet plenty of studies assume this to be the case – albeit acknowledging that it has been
'mysteriously' difficult to prove and that most people do not suffer from these symptoms
(yet experience the same changes in average circulating hormone levels).

[69] Horney (1931).

[70] Horney (1967, p 106).

[71] Horney (1967, p 106).

[72] Showalter (1993).

[73] Laws et al (1985); Parlee (1987); Chrisler and Levy (1990).

[74] Parlee (1987); Chrisler and Levy (1990); Chrisler (2002); Chrisler and Caplan (2002);
McHugh and Chrisler (2015).

[75] Laws et al (1985); Boorse (1987); Harry and Balcer (1987); Chrisler and Levy (1990);
Chrisler (2002); Chrisler and Caplan (2002).

[76] Blume (1983).

[77] Figert (1996).

[78] Figert (1996).

[79] Figert (1996).

[80] Figert (1996).

[81] Johnson (1987); Martin (1987); Laws (1990); Rittenhouse (1991); Rodin (1992); Caplan
(1995).

[82] Walker (1997, p 160).

[83] Freidson (1970).

84   Szasz (1960); Thomas and Bracken (2004).
85   Ussher (2005, 2011).
86   Chrisler (2012).
87   Dennerstein et al (2009).
88   King (2020).
89   Chang et al (1995); Yu et al (1996).
90   Chrisler (2012).
91   Rittenhouse (1991).
92   Pilver et al (2011).
93   Johnson (1987); Rodin (1992); Ussher and Perz (2013a).
94   Laws et al (1985); Rodin (1992); Ussher (2005, 2011); Ehrenreich and English (2011).
95   Halbreich et al (1982).
96   King (2020).
97   Laws et al (1985); Laws (1990).
98   Ussher (2011).
99   Martin (1987, p 121). There is also some anecdotal evidence that 'competency-based' PMS/PMDD studies are increasingly coming from countries undergoing major political and economic change, especially regarding women's rights in the workplace. For example, Ethiopia, Saudi Arabia, Iran, Turkey, China, Pakistan and India.
100   Chrisler and Levy (1990); Laws (1990, 1992); King et al (2014).
101   King (2020).
102   I have noticed a recent boom in supposedly (but not actually) empowering female health apps, products, technologies, tests and treatments. Nearly all of them blame 'hormones' for a wide variety of symptoms. The claims made by these brands are inaccurate, misleading and lacking in evidence. Knowing how much oestrogen or progesterone you have at any given moment of any day in your cycle is not going to reveal anything about your health. If any of these supplements or lifestyle changes do help with cyclic symptoms, I would imagine it is because they are anti-inflammatory and not 'hormone-balancing' as claimed. Such businesses are exploiting the fact that we are ignorant about menstrual health and often disbelieved or dismissed by our GPs, thus, forced to turn elsewhere for help. Please do not give them your money!
103   King (2020).
104   Dennerstein et al (2011); Mallia (2015).
105   RCOG (2016).

Chapter 3

1   Halbreich (2007); Knaapen and Weisz (2008); Weisz and Knaapen (2009).
2   RCOG (2016, p 81).
3   Budeiri et al (1994); Knaapen and Weisz (2008).
4   O'Brien and Ismail (2007); Weisz and Knaapen (2009).
5   Sveinsdóttir (1998).
6   Abeje and Berhanu (2019).
7   Laws (1990).
8   Martin (1987); Caplan (1995); Ussher (2005); Chrisler and Gorman (2015).
9   Laws et al (1985); Ussher (2004); Ehrenreich and English (2011).
10   Scambler and Scambler (1993); Walker (1995a); Chrisler and Caplan (2002); Ussher et al (2019).
11   Figert (1996); Walker (1997); Ussher (2005, 2011).
12   Tourangeau (1999, p 36).
13   Ruble (1977).

[14] Ruble (1977, p 292).
[15] Ruble (1977, p 292).
[16] King (2020).
[17] Pilver et al (2011); Chrisler (2012); Hawkey et al (2017); Ussher et al (2017).
[18] Scambler and Scambler (1993).
[19] Marván and Escobedo (1999, p 165).
[20] Chrisler et al (1994).
[21] Ussher and Perz (2013b, p 920).
[22] Ussher (2005); Chrisler (2012); Ussher and Perz (2013a, 2020a); McHugh and Chrisler (2015).
[23] Ussher (2005); Ussher and Perz (2020a).
[24] Ussher (2004); Ussher and Perz (2020a, 2020b).
[25] Muljat et al (2007).
[26] Kleinstäuber et al (2016).
[27] Coughlin (1990); Kuczmierczyk et al (1992); Ussher (2003); Ussher and Perz (2013a, 2013b).
[28] Ryser and Feinauer (1992); Frank et al (1993); Clayton et al (1999).
[29] Kuczmierczyk et al (1992); Ussher (2004); Chrisler et al (2014); Ussher and Perz (2017).
[30] Ussher (2003); Ussher et al (2007); Maddineshat et al (2016); Ussher and Perz (2017).
[31] Ussher and Perz (2017).
[32] Ussher and Perz (2013a).
[33] Brown and Woods (1986); Cosgrove and Riddle (2003).
[34] Ussher et al (2019).
[35] Ussher and Perz (2013a).
[36] Warner and Bancroft (1990); Warner et al (1991); Bancroft et al (1993, 1994).
[37] Logue and Moos (1986).
[38] Lee and Rittenhouse (1992).
[39] Miccio-Fonseca et al (1990); Perkonigg et al (2004).
[40] Bertone-Johnson et al (2008).
[41] For example, RCOG (2016).
[42] This is not the case. Intersectional feminist and other types of critical scholarship simply looks for evidence of political inequalities based on sex, gender, (racialised) ethnicity, sexuality and any other population characteristic potentially positioned as 'inferior'. This does not mean that researchers can simply 'invent' examples of sexism/racism/transphobia/homophobia/ableism without providing persuasive evidence. I think the myth of the hysterical female underpins this common misconception of feminist research, too.
[43] Figert (1996).
[44] Figert (1996).
[45] Wilkinson and Kitzinger (1994); Williams et al (2003); Wilson (2005); Annandale (2009).
[46] Ussher and Perz (2020b).
[47] Ussher and Perz (2020a, 2020b).
[48] Ussher and Perz (2020b).
[49] King (2020).
[50] Dennerstein et al (2011); Romans et al (2012); Mallia (2015).
[51] King (2020).
[52] Palinkas et al (2015).
[53] Cresswell and Plano Clark (2011).
[54] Dennerstein et al (2011); Quintana-Zinn et al (2017).
[55] Cortese and Brown (1989); Dennerstein et al (2010); Ussher and Perz (2013a).

[56] Schmelzer et al (2015); de Carvalho et al (2018).
[57] Marván and Escobedo (1999); Dennerstein et al (2011).
[58] Chrisler (2012); Ussher et al (2012); Hawkey et al (2017).
[59] Johnson (1987); Dennerstein et al (2010).
[60] Hawkey et al (2017).
[61] Despite engaging with some highly marginalised communities, it was only university-educated 'patients' who volunteered to participate. Without further investigation (beyond the scope of my study), this could indicate any of several things previously identified by researchers: That knowledge of, attribution of experiences to, and help-seeking behaviour for, PMS may vary with socioeconomic status and/or educational attainment (Petta et al, 2010; Dennerstein et al, 2011), that university-educated individuals may be more able to attend health-related community meetings or talks, or to volunteer in general (Parboteeah et al, 2004; McGarvey et al, 2020), that associated stigma may prevent some people from wanting to publicly discuss their (pre)menstrual experiences (Johnston-Robledo and Chrisler, 2013; Hawkey et al, 2017), or that my relatively privileged embodied status as a six-foot tall, White, middle-class, university-affiliated researcher put off some potential participants (Sharma et al, 2009).
[62] Sims-Schouten and Riley (2014, p 57).
[63] Fairclough (2014).
[64] Glaser and Strauss (1967).
[65] Corbin and Strauss (2008).
[66] Sims-Schouten and Riley (2014).
[67] Sims-Schouten and Riley (2014).
[68] Tan et al (2017); Cohen (2020).
[69] Mallia (2015).
[70] Dennerstein et al (2011).
[71] Romans et al (2012).
[72] Gold et al (2016).
[73] https://reshare.ukdataservice.ac.uk/855486/
[74] Knight and colleagues found that the dismissal of patient concerns was a contributing factor in disproportionate numbers of racialised British women dying in childbirth in the UK (Knight et al, 2020).
[75] https://beta.ukdataservice.ac.uk/datacatalogue/studies/study?id=855486

Chapter 4

[1] RCOG (2016).
[2] Dennerstein et al (2011); Mallia (2015).
[3] Dennerstein et al (2011).
[4] Thong et al (2017); Orhan et al (2018).
[5] Chrisler (2012).
[6] Walley-Jean (2009); Ashley (2014).
[7] Wandner et al (2012); Hoffman et al (2016); Mende-Siedlecki et al (2019).
[8] FitzGerald and Hurst (2017); Hewes et al (2018); Knight et al (2020).
[9] RCOG (2016).
[10] APA (2013).
[11] Romans et al (2012).
[12] RCOG (2016).
[13] Romans et al (2012).
[14] APA (1994).
[15] King (2020).

[16] Romans et al (2012).

[17] Hoffmann and Tarzian (2001); Ashley (2014); Hoffman et al (2016); Knight et al (2020).

Chapter 5

[1] Scambler and Scambler (1993).

[2] Martin (1987); Ussher (2005); Ehrenreich and English (2011); Khamlichi (2016).

[3] Figert (1996); Chrisler and Caplan (2002); Ussher (2005).

[4] Romans et al (2012); Mallia (2015).

[5] Woods et al (1992); Scambler and Scambler (1993); O'Flynn and Britten (2000); Santer et al (2008).

[6] Dennerstein et al (2011).

[7] Dennerstein et al (2011).

[8] Ohde et al (2008); Zhou et al (2010).

[9] ACOG (2018).

[10] ACOG (2018).

[11] ACOG (2018).

Chapter 6

[1] At the time of interview, three of the biomedical experts were involved in the development of a 'PMDD-specific' drug designed to reduce circulating levels of allopregnanolone (a metabolite of progesterone). After a promising pilot study, the drug was found to be only as effective as placebo in a larger controlled trial, first reported in April 2020 (IAPMD, 2021). At time of interview (November 2019 to March 2020), some participants were likely to have been influenced by the pilot study results. Interestingly, a subsequent 're-analysis' of the data, and retrospective change in methodology (measuring changes over nine premenstrual days rather than five) found a statistically significant difference between a low dosage of the drug versus placebo response – but the clinical difference in symptom expression remained very small (Bäckström et al, 2021). The fact that the data had to be 're-analysed' in the first place suggests 'data dredging' (the trawling of a data set to find any and all 'statistically significant' relationships between factors, regardless of the original hypothesis or proposed analytical metholodgy). This is not good scientific practice.

[2] Backstrom et al (1983); Rubinow et al (1988); Rubinow and Schmidt (1995); Schmidt et al (1998).

[3] Carothers and Reis (2013) found no difference between men and women (n=13,000) in relation to the main psychological characteristics described in John Gray's best-selling book *Men Are from Mars, Women Are from Venus*. Like most 'sex differences', despite there being some variation in average values, the distributions overlapped so much that a categorical sex-based distinction was not meaningful.

[4] The proportion of the UK female population of reproductive age (between 12 and 52 years old) is approximately 51 per cent, based on 2018 population data (ONS, 2020).

[5] Romans et al (2012); Mallia (2015).

[6] Ussher (1989, 2011); Ussher and Perz (2013b).

[7] Laws et al (1985); Martin (1987); Ussher (2005).

[8] Romans et al (2012); Mallia (2015).

[9] Sexist pseudo-scientific articles within evolutionary psychology and biology have attracted media attention in recent years. One deeply problematic study concluded that women experience oestrus/conspicuous ovulation (even though human ovulation is concealed and notoriously difficult to detect) because nine lap dancers received more tips from male punters around this phase of their menstrual cycle (Miller et al, 2007). The study did not consider factors such as pay day timing, cyclical changes in body confidence, or the fact

that men paying lap dancers was hardly a natural human interaction or even a relevant proxy for 'mating attraction' (particularly from the point of view of the dancers). Others have implied that women are 'more inclined to cheat on their long-term male partners' around ovulation, which assumes that women have no or reduced agency on account of their 'hormones' (Jones et al, 2005). In short, unscientific and demonstrably sexist research continues to attract funding and publication, even in supposedly quality journals.

[10] Dennerstein et al (2011).

[11] Van Tilburg et al (2003); Vingerhoets et al (2007).

[12] Sharman et al (2019).

[13] Ussher (2004, 2005); Ussher and Perz (2020a).

[14] Ehrenreich and English (2011).

[15] RCOG (2016).

[16] Dennerstein et al (2011).

[17] Greene and Dalton (1953).

[18] Budeiri et al (1994).

[19] Sveinsdóttir and Bäckström (2000); Halbreich et al (2003); Gehlert et al (2009); Nowosielski et al (2010).

[20] Mallia (2015, pp 104–105).

[21] Mallia (2015, pp 94–102).

[22] Ternhag et al (2005).

[23] Zukerstein (2015).

Chapter 7

[1] Emera et al (2012).

[2] Greer (1999); Manicom (2010).

[3] Delaney et al (1976); Dunnavant and Roberts (2013); Johnston-Robledo and Chrisler (2013).

[4] Marván and Escobedo (1999); Read et al (2014).

[5] Tingle and Vora (2018); Chandra-Mouli and Patel (2020).

[6] Craner et al (2014).

[7] This finding is largely due to the average age of the expert group (over 60 years old). PMS only became a well-known societal/biomedical label in the early 1980s, when most of the group were already adults.

[8] Edwards et al (2014).

[9] Bendtzen et al (2003).

[10] King (2024).

[11] Walker (1995a).

[12] Sims-Schouten et al (2007).

Chapter 8

[1] Southam and Gonzaga (1965); Maybin et al (2011); Critchley et al (2020).

[2] Fothergill (1899); Southam and Gonzaga (1965); Finn (1986); Blackman (2001).

[3] Birke (1999); Roberts (2007); Annandale (2009).

[4] Caplan (1995); Figert (1996); Ussher (2005).

[5] Knight et al (2020).

[6] Hoffmann and Tarzian (2001); Weisse et al (2001).

[7] Hyun et al (2017); Asthana et al (2018).

[8] For example, RCOG (2016).

[9] For example, RCOG (2016).

[10] Marván and Escobedo (1999); Ussher and Perz (2013b); Read et al (2014).

[11] McFarlane et al (1988); McFarlane and Williams (1994); Kiesner et al (2020); Schmalenberger et al (2021).

[12] King (2024).

[13] I am talking about addiction-related behaviours usually relating to opiate prescriptions, which are not typically relevant for UK-based healthcare or menstrual cycle-related symptoms. A prescription for anti-inflammatory medications for use around menstruation is of very low risk for abuse. I am certainly *not* including subjective impressions of 'attention-seeking' or suspected mental health issues, because it is perfectly possible for someone with challenging behaviours to also be experiencing physical pain.

References

Abeje, A. and Berhanu, Z. (2019) 'Premenstrual syndrome and factors associated with it among secondary and preparatory school students in Debremarkos town, north-west Ethiopia, 2016', *BMC Research Notes*, 12(1), Article 535.

Abrams, E.T. and Miller, E.M. (2011) 'The roles of the immune system in women's reproduction: Evolutionary constraints and life history trade-offs', *American Journal of Physical Anthropology*, 146(S53), pp 134–154.

ACOG (2018) 'ACOG committee opinion no. 760: Dysmenorrhea and endometriosis in the adolescent', *Obstetrics and Gynecology*, 132(6), pp 249–258.

Angeli, A., Lainé, F., Lavenu, A., Ropert, M., Lacut, K., Gissot, V., et al (2016) 'Joint model of iron and hepcidin during the menstrual cycle in healthy women', *AAPS Journal*, 18(2), pp 490–504.

Annandale, E. (2009) *Women's Health and Social Change*. London and New York: Routledge.

APA (1987) *Diagnostic and Statistical Manual of Mental Disorders (DSM III R)*. 3rd revised edn. South Dartmouth: American Psychiatric Association.

APA (1994) *Diagnostic and Statistical Manual of Mental Disorders (DSM IV)*. 4th edn. South Dartmouth: American Psychiatric Association.

APA (2013) *Diagnostic and Statistical Manual of Mental Disorders (DSM V)*. 5th edn. South Dartmouth: American Psychiatric Association.

Asbring, P. and Närvänen, A. (2002) 'Women's experiences of stigma in relation to chronic fatigue syndrome and fibromyalgia', *Qualitative Health Research*, 12(2), pp 148–160.

Ashley, W. (2014) 'The angry black woman: The impact of pejorative stereotypes on psychotherapy with black women', *Social Work in Public Health*, 29(1), pp 27–34.

As-Sanie, S., Black, R., Giudice, L.C., Valbrun, T.G., Gupta, J., Jones, B., et al (2019) 'Assessing research gaps and unmet needs in endometriosis', *American Journal of Obstetrics and Gynecology*, 221(2), pp 86–94.

Asthana, S., Moon, G., Gibson, A., Bailey, T., Hewson, P. and Dibben, C. (2018) 'Inequity in cardiovascular care in the English National Health Service (NHS): A scoping review of the literature', *Health & Social Care in the Community*, 26(3), pp 259–272.

Ávila, L.A. and Terra, J.R. (2012) 'Hysteria and its metamorphoses', *Revista Latinoamericana de Psicopatologia Fundamental*, 15(1), pp 27–41.

Avis, N.E., Crawford, S.L. and Green, R. (2018) 'Vasomotor symptoms across the menopause transition: Differences among women', *Obstetrics and Gynecology Clinics of North America*, 316(4), pp 629–640.

Bäckström, T., Sanders, D., Leask, R., Davidson, D., Warner, P. and Bancroft, J. (1983) 'Mood, sexuality, hormones, and the menstrual cycle: Hormone levels and their relationship to the premenstrual syndrome', *Psychosomatic Medicine*, 45(6), pp 503–507.

Bäckström, T., Ekberg, K., Hirschberg, A.L., Bixo, M., Epperson, C.N., Briggs, P., et al (2021) 'A randomized, double-blind study on efficacy and safety of sepranolone in premenstrual dysphoric disorder', *Psychoneuroendocrinology*, 133(1), Article 105426.

Balik, G., Ustüner, I., Kağitci, M. and Sahin, F.K. (2014) 'Is there a relationship between mood disorders and dysmenorrhea?', *Journal of Pediatric and Adolescent Gynecology*, 27(6), pp 371–374.

Bancroft, J., Williamson, L., Warner, P., Rennie, D. and Smith, S.K. (1993) 'Perimenstrual complaints in women complaining of PMS, menorrhagia, and dysmenorrhea: Toward a dismantling of the premenstrual syndrome', *Psychosomatic Medicine*, 55(2), pp 133–145.

Bancroft, J., Rennie, D. and Warner, P. (1994) 'Vulnerability to perimenstrual mood change: The relevance of a past history of depressive disorder', *Psychosomatic Medicine*, 56(3), pp 225–231.

Barabás, K., Szabó-Meleg, E. and Ábrahám, I.M. (2020) 'Effect of inflammation on female gonadotropin-releasing hormone (GnRH) neurons: Mechanisms and consequences', *International Journal of Molecular Sciences*, 21(2), Article 529.

Barrett, K.E., Barman, S., Yuan, J. and Brooks, H. (2019) *Ganong's Review of Medical Physiology*. 7th edn. New York: McGraw-Hill.

BBC News Online (2020) 'Vaginal mesh: UK government told to apologise after "damning" review'. Available at: https://www.bbc.co.uk/news/uk-wales-53323780

BBC Newsround (2020) 'What do medical conditions look like on darker skin?', August. Available at: https://www.bbc.co.uk/newsround/53448162

Behboudi-Gandevani, S., Hariri, F.Z. and Moghaddam-Banaem, L. (2018) 'The effect of omega 3 fatty acid supplementation on premenstrual syndrome and health-related quality of life: A randomized clinical trial', *Journal of Psychosomatic Obstetrics and Gynecology*, 39(4), pp 266–272.

Bellei, E., Rustichelli, C., Bergamini, S., Monari, E., Baraldi, C., Lo Castro, F., et al (2020) 'Proteomic serum profile in menstrual-related and post menopause migraine', *Journal of Pharmaceutical and Biomedical Analysis*, 184(113165), pp 1–8.

Bellofiore, N. and Evans, J. (2019) 'Monkeys, mice and menses: The bloody anomaly of the spiny mouse', *Journal of Assisted Reproduction and Genetics*, 36(5), pp 811–817.

Bendtzen, K., Hansen, P.R. and Rieneck, K. (2003) 'Spironolactone inhibits production of proinflammatory cytokines, including tumour necrosis factor-α and interferon-γ and has potential in the treatment of arthritis', *Clinical and Experimental Immunology*, 134(1), pp 151–158.

Bertone-Johnson, E.R. (2016) 'Chronic inflammation and premenstrual syndrome: A missing link found?', *Journal of Women's Health*, 25(9), pp 857–858.

Bertone-Johnson, E.R., Hankinson, S.E., Johnson, S.R. and Manson, J.E. (2008) 'Cigarette smoking and the development of premenstrual syndrome', *American Journal of Epidemiology*, 168(8), pp 938–945.

Bertone-Johnson, E.R., Ronnenberg, A.G., Houghton, S.C., Nobles, C., Zagarins, S.E., Takashima-Uebelhoer, B.B., et al (2014) 'Association of inflammation markers with menstrual symptom severity and premenstrual syndrome in young women', *Human Reproduction*, 29(9), pp 1987–1994.

Birke, L. (1999) *Feminism and the Biological Body*. Edinburgh: Edinburgh University Press.

Blackman, H. (2001) *Women, Savages and Other Animals: The Comparative Physiology of Reproduction, 1850–1914*. Thesis submitted to the University of Manchester. https://isni.org/isni/0000000426936675

Blume, E. (1983) 'Premenstrual syndromes, depression linked', *JAMA: The Journal of the American Medical Association*, 249(21), pp 2864–2866.

Bobel, C. (2010) *New Blood: Third-Wave Feminism and the Politics of Menstruation*. Piscataway: Rutgers University Press.

Bobel, C. (2019) *The Managed Body*. New York: Springer International.

Boorse, C. (1987) 'Premenstrual syndrome and criminal responsibility', in G.E. Ginsburg and B.F. Carter (eds) *Premenstrual Syndrome*. Boston: Springer US, pp 81–124.

Boron, W.F. and Bouldaep, E.L. (2017) *Boron & Boulpaep Medical Physiology*. 3rd edn. Philadelphia: Elsevier.

Brosens, J.J., Bennett, P.R., Abrahams, V.M., Ramhorst, R., Coomarasamy, A., Quenby, S., et al (2022) 'Maternal selection of human embryos in early gestation: Insights from recurrent miscarriage', *Seminars in Cell & Developmental Biology*, 131, pp 14–24.

Brown, M.A. and Woods, N.F. (1986) 'Sex role orientation, sex typing, occupational traditionalism, and perimenstrual symptoms', *Health Care for Women International*, 7(1–2), pp 25–37.

Brulin-Solignac, D., de Jésus, A., Defanti De Agostinho, C. and Bouchard, J.-P. (2021) 'Hysteria: History of a concept and its clinical reality', *Soins. Psychiatrie*, 42(335), pp 12–17.

Budeiri, D.J., Wan Po, A.-L. and Dornan, J.C. (1994) 'Clinical trials of treatments of premenstrual syndrome: Entry criteria and scales for measuring treatment outcomes', *BJOG: An International Journal of Obstetrics and Gynaecology*, 101(8), pp 689–695.

Bull, J.R., Rowland, S.P., Scherwitzl, E.B., Scherwitzl, R., Danielsson, K.G. and Harper, J. (2019) 'Real-world menstrual cycle characteristics of more than 600,000 menstrual cycles', *npj Digital Medicine*, 2(1), Article 83.

Cannon, C. and Nasrallah, H.A. (2019) 'A focus on postpartum depression among African American women: A literature review', *Annals of Clinical Psychiatry: Official Journal of the American Academy of Clinical Psychiatrists*, 31(2), pp 138–143.

Caplan, P.J. (1995) *They Say You're Crazy: How the World's Most Powerful Psychiatrists Decide Who's Normal.* Boston: Da Capo Press.

Cappellini, M.D., Musallam, K.M. and Taher, A.T. (2020) 'Iron deficiency anaemia revisited', *Journal of Internal Medicine*, 287(2), pp 153–170.

Carothers, B.J. and Reis, H.T. (2013) 'Men and women are from earth: Examining the latent structure of gender', *Journal of Personality and Social Psychology*, 104(2), pp 385–407.

Casimiri, V. and Psychoyos, A. (1981) 'Embryo-endometrial relationships during implantation', in J. de Brux, R. Mortel and J.P. Gautray (eds) *The Endometrium.* Boston: Springer US, pp 63–79.

CGP (2017) *Grade 9–1 GCSE Biology Edexcel Complete Revision & Practice with Online Edition.* Available at: https://www.cgpbooks.co.uk/second ary-books/gcse/science/biology/bes41-grade-9-1-gcse-biology-edexcel

CGP (2021) *GCSE Biology AQA Complete Revision & Practice includes Online Ed, Videos & Quizzes.* Available at: https://www.cgpbooks.co.uk/secondary-books/gcse/science/biology/bas46-gcse-biology-aqa-complete-revision

Chandra-Mouli, V. and Patel, S.V. (2020) 'Mapping the knowledge and understanding of menarche, menstrual hygiene and menstrual health among adolescent girls in low- and middle-income countries', in C. Bobel, I.T. Winkler, B. Fahs, K.A. Hasson, E.A. Kissling and T.-A. Roberts (eds) *The Palgrave Handbook of Critical Menstruation Studies.* Singapore: Springer Singapore, pp 609–636.

Chang, A.M., Holroyd, E. and Chau, J.P.C. (1995) 'Premenstrual syndrome in employed Chinese women in Hong Kong', *Health Care for Women International*, 16(6), pp 551–561.

Charkoudian, N., Hart, E., Barnes, J.N. and Joyner, M.J. (2017) 'Autonomic control of body temperature and blood pressure: Influences of female sex hormones', *Clinical Autonomic Research*, 27(3), pp 149–155.

Chocano-Bedoya, P., Manson, J.E., Hankinson, S.E., Johnson, S.R., Chasan-Taber, L., Ronnenberg, A.G., et al (2013) 'Intake of selected minerals and risk of premenstrual syndrome', *American Journal of Epidemiology*, 177(10), pp 1118–1127.

Chrisler, J. (2002) 'Hormone hostages: The cultural legacy of PMS as a legal defense', in L.H. Collins, M.R. Dunlap and J.C. Chrisler (eds) *Charting a New Course for Feminist Psychology*, Westport: Praeger, pp 238–252.

Chrisler, J. (2012) 'PMS as a culture-bound syndrome', in J. Chrisler, C. Golden and P.D. Rozee (eds) *Lectures on the Psychology of Women*. 4th edn. Long Grove: Waveland Press, pp 155–171.

Chrisler, J. and Levy, K. (1990) 'The media construct a menstrual monster: A content analysis of PMS articles in the popular press', *Women & Health*, 16(2), pp 89–104.

Chrisler, J. and Caplan, P. (2002) 'The strange case of Dr. Jekyll and Ms. Hyde: How PMS became a cultural phenomenon and a psychiatric disorder', *Annual Review of Sex Research*, 13, pp 274–306.

Chrisler, J. and Gorman, J. (2015) 'The medicalization of women's moods: Premenstrual syndrome and premenstrual dysphoric disorder', in M.C. McHugh and J. Chrisler (eds) *The Wrong Prescription for Women: How Medicine and Media Create a 'Need' for Treatments, Drugs, and Surgery*. Santa Barbara: Praeger, pp 77–98.

Chrisler, J., Johnston, I.K., Champagne, N.M. and Preston, K.E. (1994) 'Menstrual joy: The construct and its consequences', *Psychology of Women Quarterly*, 18(3), pp 375–387.

Chrisler, J., Gorman, J. and Streckfuss, L. (2014) 'Self-silencing, perfectionism, dualistic discourse, loss of control, and the experience of premenstrual syndrome', *Women's Reproductive Health*, 1(2), pp 138–152.

Christodoulakos, G., Augoulea, A., Lambrinoudaki, I., Sioulas, V. and Creatsas, G. (2009) 'Pathogenesis of endometriosis: The role of defective "immunosurveillance"', *The European Journal of Contraceptive and Reproductive Healthcare*, 12(3), pp 194–202.

Clark, J., Hurley, R., Ladher, N. and Jarvies, D. (2023) 'What next for decolonising health and medicine?', *BMJ*, 383, Article 2302.

Clayton, A.H., Clavet, G.J., McGarvey, E.L., Warnock, J.K. and Weiss, K. (1999) 'Assessment of sexual functioning during the menstrual cycle', *Journal of Sex & Marital Therapy*, 25(4), pp 281–291.

Cohen, I. (2020) 'Menstruation and religion: Developing a critical menstrual studies approach', in C. Bobel, I.T. Winkler, B. Fahs, K.A. Hasson, E.A. Kissling and T.-A. Roberts (eds) *The Palgrave Handbook of Critical Menstruation Studies*. Singapore: Springer, pp 115–129.

Collao, N., Rada, I., Francaux, M., Deldicque, L. and Zbinden-Foncea, H. (2020) 'Anti-inflammatory effect of exercise mediated by toll-like receptor regulation in innate immune cells – a review', *International Reviews of Immunology*, 39(2), pp 39–52.

Collins, S., Arulkumaran, S., Hayes, K., Jackson, S. and Impey, L. (2013) *Oxford Handbook of Obstetrics and Gynaecology*. Oxford: Oxford University Press.

Constanzo, L. (2018a) *BRS Physiology*. 7th edn. Philadelphia: Wolters Kluwer.

Constanzo, L. (2018b) *Constanzo's Physiology*. 6th edn. New York: Elsevier.

Corbin, J. and Strauss, A. (2008) *Basics of Qualitative Research (3rd ed.): Techniques and Procedures for Developing Grounded Theory*. London: SAGE.

Cordage, S.P. (1684) *An Essay of the Pathology of the Brain and Nervous Stock in which Convulsive Diseases are Treated, by Thomas Willis*. English translation edited by S.P. Cordage. London: Dring, Leigh & Harper.

Cortese, J. and Brown, M.A. (1989) 'Coping responses of men whose partners experience premenstrual symptomatology', *Journal of Obstetric, Gynecologic & Neonatal Nursing*, 18(5), pp 405–412.

Cosgrove, L. and Riddle, B. (2003) 'Constructions of femininity and experiences of menstrual distress', *Women & Health*, 38(3), pp 37–58.

Coughlin, P.C. (1990) 'Premenstrual syndrome: How marital satisfaction and role choice affect symptom severity', *Social Work (United States)*, 35(4), pp 351–355.

Craner, J.R., Sigmon, S.T. and McGillicuddy, M.L. (2014) 'Does a disconnect occur between research and practice for premenstrual dysphoric disorder (PMDD) diagnostic procedures?', *Women and Health*, 54(3), pp 232–244.

Cresswell, J.W. and Plano Clark, V.L. (2011) *Designing and Conducting Mixed Methods Research*. 2nd edn. London: SAGE.

Critchley, H.D. and Garfinkel, S.N. (2017) 'Interoception and emotion', *Current Opinion in Psychology*, 17, pp 7–14.

Critchley, H.D., Babayev, E., Bulun, S.E., Clark, S., Garcia-Grau, I., Gregersen, P.K., et al (2020) 'Menstruation: Science and society', *American Journal of Obstetrics and Gynecology*, 223(5), pp 624–664.

Dalton, K. (1964) *The Premenstrual Syndrome*. London: Heinemann.

Dalton, K. (1969) *The Menstrual Cycle*. Harmondsworth: Penguin.

de Beauvoir, S. (2010) *The Second Sex*. Translated by C. Borde and S. Malovany-Chevallier. London: Vintage.

De Benedictis, S. (2023) 'Periods of austerity: The emergence of "period poverty" in UK news media', *European Journal of Cultural Studies*, 26(6), pp 880–896.

de Carvalho, A.B., de Azevedo Cardoso, T., Mondin, T.C., da Silva, R., de Mattos Souza, L.D., da Silva Magalhães, P.V., et al (2018) 'Prevalence and factors associated with Premenstrual Dysphoric Disorder: A community sample of young adult women', *Psychiatry Research*, 268, pp 42–45.

Delaney, J., Lupton, J. and Toth, E. (1976) *The Curse: A Cultural History of Menstruation*. Champaign: University of Illinois Press.

DeLuca, R.S. (2017) *The Hormone Myth: How Junk Science, Gender Politics, & Lies about PMS Keep Women Down*. Oakland: New Harbinger.

Dennerstein, L., Lehert, P., Bäckström, T.C. and Heinemann, K. (2009) 'Premenstrual symptoms – severity, duration and typology: An international cross-sectional study', *Menopause International*, 15(3), pp 120–126.

Dennerstein, L., Lehert, P., Bäckström, T.C. and Heinemann, K. (2010) 'The effect of premenstrual symptoms on activities of daily life', *Fertility and Sterility*, 94(3), pp 1059–1064.

Dennerstein, L., Lehert, P. and Heinemann, K. (2011) 'Global study of women's experiences of premenstrual symptoms and their effects on daily life', *Menopause International*, 17(3), pp 88–95.

Descartes, R. (1637) *Discours de la méthode: pour bien conduire sa raison et chercher la vérité dans les sciences*. Leiden: Jan Maire.

Devereux, C. (2014) 'Hysteria, feminism, and gender revisited: The case of the second wave', *English Studies in Canada*, 40(1), pp 19–45.

Dionisie, V., Filip, G.A., Manea, M.C., Manea, M. and Riga, S. (2021) 'The anti-inflammatory role of SSRI and SNRI in the treatment of depression: A review of human and rodent research studies', *Inflammopharmacology*, 29(1), pp 75–90.

Duby, G. and Perrot, M. (1993) *A History of Women in the West; III. Renaissance and Enlightenment Paradoxes*. Cambridge, MA: Harvard University Press.

Dugan, C., MacLean, B., Cabolis, K., Abeysiri, S., Khong, A., Sajic, M., et al (2021) 'The misogyny of iron deficiency', *Anaesthesia*, 76(S4), pp 56–62.

Dunnavant, N.C. and Roberts, T.-A. (2013) 'Restriction and renewal, pollution and power, constraint and community: The paradoxes of religious women's experiences of menstruation', *Sex Roles*, 68(1–2), pp 121–131.

Edwards, P.K., O'Mahoney, J. and Vincent, S. (2014) *Studying Organizations Using Critical Realism: A Practical Guide*. Oxford: Oxford University Press.

Ehrenreich, B. and English, D. (2011) *Complaints and Disorders: The Sexual Politics of Sickness*. 2nd edn. New York: The Feminist Press.

Emera, D., Romero, R. and Wagner, G. (2012) 'The evolution of menstruation: A new model for genetic assimilation', *BioEssays*, 34(1), pp 26–35.

Espey, L. (1980) 'Ovulation as an inflammatory reaction: A hypothesis', *Biology of Reproduction*, 22(1), pp 73–106.

Fairclough, N. (2014) *Critical Language Awareness*. 2nd edn. London: Taylor & Francis.

Farland, L.V., Shah, D.K., Kvaskoff, M., Zondervan, K.T. and Missmer, S.A. (2017) 'Epidemiological and clinical risk factors for endometriosis', in T. D'Hooghe (ed) *Biomarkers for Endometriosis: State of the Art*. Cham: Springer, pp 95–121.

Federici, S. (2004) *Caliban and the Witch*. 1st edn. Brooklyn: Autonomedia.

Figert, A. (1996) *Women and the Ownership of PMS: The Structuring of a Psychiatric Disorder*. New York: Aldine De Gruyter.

Finn, C.A. (1986) 'Implantation, menstruation and inflammation', *Biological Reviews of the Cambridge Philosophical Society*, 61(4), pp 313–328.

FitzGerald, C. and Hurst, S. (2017) 'Implicit bias in healthcare professionals: A systematic review', *BMC Medical Ethics*, 18(1), Article 19.

Fothergill, W.E. (1899) 'The function of decidual cells', *Edinburgh Medical Journal*, 5, pp 265–273.

Fraisse, G. (1994) *Reason's Muse: Sexual Difference and the Birth of Democracy*. Chicago: University of Chicago Press.

Frank, B., Dixon, D.N. and Grosz, H.J. (1993) 'Conjoint monitoring of symptoms of premenstrual syndrome: Impact on marital satisfaction', *Journal of Counseling Psychology*, 40(1), pp 109–114.

Frank, R. (1929) *The Female Sex Hormone*. Springfield: Charles C Thomas.

Frank, R. (1931) 'The hormonal causes of premenstrual tension', *Archives of Neurology Psychiatry*, 26(5), pp 1053–1057.

Fraser, I., Warner, P. and Marantos, P. (2001) 'Estimating menstrual blood loss in women with normal and excessive menstrual fluid volume', *Obstetrics and Gynecology*, 98(5), pp 806–814.

Freidson, E. (1970) *Profession of Medicine: A Study of the Sociology of Applied Knowledge*. Chicago: University of Chicago Press.

Freud, S. and Breuer, J. (1895) *Studies in Hysteria*. English translation. Harmondsworth: Penguin.

Fricker, M. and Hornsby, J. (2001) 'The Cambridge companion to feminism in philosophy', *Ethics*, 112(1), pp 145–148.

Friedan, B. (1963) *The Feminine Mystique*. Harmondsworth: Penguin.

Gao, M., Gao, D., Sun, H., Cheng, X., An, L. and Qiao, M. (2021) 'Trends in research related to premenstrual syndrome and premenstrual dysphoric disorder from 1945 to 2018: A bibliometric analysis', *Frontiers in Public Health*, 9, Article 596128.

Gehlert, S., Song, I.H., Chang, C.-H. and Hartlage, S.A. (2009) 'The prevalence of premenstrual dysphoric disorder in a randomly selected group of urban and rural women', *Psychological Medicine*, 39(1), pp 129–136.

Gilman, S.L., King, H., Porter, R., Rousseau, G.S. and Showalter, E. (1993) *Hysteria beyond Freud*. Berkeley: University of California Press.

Glaser, B. and Strauss, A. (1967) *The Discovery of Grounded Theory*. London: Weidenfeld & Nicolson.

Gold, E., Wells, C. and Rasor, M. (2016) 'The association of inflammation with premenstrual symptoms', *Journal of Women's Health*, 25(9), pp 865–874.

Graziottin, A. and Serafini, A. (2016) 'Perimenstrual asthma: From pathophysiology to treatment strategies', *Multidisciplinary Respiratory Medicine*, 11(1), Article 30.

Greene, R. and Dalton, K. (1953) 'The premenstrual syndrome', *BMJ*, 1(4818), pp 1007–1014.

Greer, G. (1999) *The Whole Woman*. 1st edn. New York: Doubleday.

Grose, A. (2016) *Hysteria Today*. Oxford: Routledge.

Gunter, J. (2024) *Blood: The Science, Medicine, and Mythology of Menstruation*. London: Little Brown Book Group.

Hafiz, S.P., Barnes, N.L.P. and Kirwan, C.C. (2018) 'Clinical management of idiopathic mastalgia: A systematic review', *Journal of Primary Health Care*, 10(4), pp 312–323.

Halbreich, U. (2007) 'The diagnosis of PMS/PMDD: The current debate', in P.M.S. O'Brien, A.J. Rapkin and P.J. Schmidt (eds) *The Premenstrual Syndromes: PMS and PMDD*. Boca Raton: CRC Press, pp 9–19.

Halbreich, U., Endicott, J., Schacht, S. and Nee, J. (1982) 'The diversity of premenstrual changes as reflected in the Premenstrual Assessment Form', *Acta Psychiatrica Scandinavica*, 65, pp 46–65.

Halbreich, U., Borenstein, J., Pearlstein, T. and Kahn, L.S. (2003) 'The prevalence, impairment, impact, and burden of premenstrual dysphoric disorder (PMS/PMDD)', *Psychoneuroendocrinology*, 28, pp 1–23.

Hall, J.E. and Hall, M.E. (2021) *Guyton and Hall: Textbook of Medical Physiology*. 14th edn. New York: Elsevier.

Hancock, A., Weeks, A.D. and Lavender, D.T. (2015) 'Is accurate and reliable blood loss estimation the "crucial step" in early detection of postpartum haemorrhage: An integrative review of the literature', *BMC Pregnancy Childbirth*, 15, pp 1–9.

Harrison, N.A. (2017) 'Brain structures implicated in inflammation-associated depression', in R. Dantzer and L. Capuron (eds) *Inflammation-Associated Depression: Evidence, Mechanisms and Implications*. Cham: Springer International, pp 221–248.

Harry, B. and Balcer, C.M. (1987) 'Menstruation and crime: A critical review of the literature from the clinical criminology perspective', *Behavioral Sciences & the Law*, 5(3), pp 307–321.

Hawkey, A.J., Ussher, J.M., Perz, J. and Metusela, C. (2017) 'Experiences and constructions of menarche and menstruation among migrant and refugee women', *Qualitative Health Research*, 27(10), pp 1473–1490.

Heffner, L.J. and Schust, D.J. (2014) *Human Reproduction at a Glance*. 4th edn. Oxford: Wiley-Blackwell.

Hess, R.A., Bunick, D., Lee, K.-H., Bahr, J., Taylor, J.A., Korach, K.S., et al (1997) 'A role for oestrogens in the male reproductive system', *Nature*, 390(6659), pp 509–512.

Hewes, H.A., Dai, M., Mann, N.C., Baca, T. and Taillac, P. (2018) 'Prehospital pain management: Disparity by age and race', *Prehospital Emergency Care*, 22(2), pp 189–197.

Hippocrates of Cos (2018) *Diseases of Women, Volume I*. Edited by P. Potter. Cambridge, MA: Harvard University Press.

Hoffman, K.M., Trawalter, S., Axt, J.R. and Oliver, M.N. (2016) 'Racial bias in pain assessment and treatment recommendations, and false beliefs about biological differences between blacks and whites', *Proceedings of the National Academy of Sciences of the United States of America*, 113(16), pp 4296–4301.

Hoffmann, D.E. and Tarzian, A.J. (2001) 'The girl who cried pain: a bias against women in the treatment of pain', *Journal of Law, Medicine and Ethics*, 29, pp 13–27.

Horney, K. (1931) 'Die prämenstruellen Verstimmungen' ['Premenstrual tensions'], *Zeitschrift für Psychoanalytische Pädagogik*, 5(1), pp 1–7.

Horney, K. (1967) *Feminine Psychology* (English translation). Edited by H. Kelman. New York: London: W. Norton & Company.

Howard, R.D. and Howard, R.S. (2022) 'Shell shock: The response of UK neurology', *European Neurology*, 85(2), pp 162–168.

Hyun, K.K., Redfern, J., Patel, A., Peiris, D., Brieger, D., Sullivan, D., et al (2017) 'Gender inequalities in cardiovascular risk factor assessment and management in primary healthcare', *Heart*, 103(7), pp 492–498.

IAPMD (2021) *What Happened to the PMDD-specific Treatment (Sepranalone) that was being Developed?* Available at: https://faq.iapmd.org/en/articles/4005826-what-happened-to-the-pmdd-specific-treatment-sepranalone-that-was-being-developed

Jarvis, G.E. (2016) 'Estimating limits for natural human embryo mortality', *F1000Research*, 5, Article 2083.

Jefferson, G. (2004) 'Glossary of transcript symbols with an introduction', in G. Lerner (ed) *Conversation Analysis: Studies from the First Generation*. Amsterdam: John Benjamins, pp 13–31.

Johnson, S. (1987) 'The epidemiology and social impact of premenstrual symptoms', *Clinical Obstetrics and Gynecology*, 30(2), pp 367–376.

Johnson, T.M. (1987) 'Premenstrual syndrome as a Western culture-specific disorder', *Culture, Medicine and Psychiatry*, 11(3), pp 337–356.

Johnston-Robledo, I. and Chrisler, J. (2013) 'The menstrual mark: Menstruation as social stigma', *Sex Roles*, 68(1–2), pp 9–18.

Jones, B.C., Little, A.C., Boothroyd, L., Debruine, L.M., Feinberg, D.R., Law Smith, M.J., et al (2005) 'Commitment to relationships and preferences for femininity and apparent health in faces are strongest on days of the menstrual cycle when progesterone level is high', *Hormones and Behavior*, 48(3), pp 283–290.

Jones, R.E. and Lopez, K.H. (2013) *Human Reproductive Biology: Fourth Edition*. London: Elsevier.

Khamlichi, S. (2016) *Medicalising Menstruation: The Case of Premenstrual Dysphoric Disorder and DSM V*. PhD thesis submitted to the University of East London. Available at https://repository.uel.ac.uk/item/85vv7

Khan, S. (2023) '£1m payout after avoidable mesh surgery led to complications', *BBC News Online*. Available at: https://www.bbc.co.uk/news/uk-england-coventry-warwickshire-67407968

Kiesner, J., Eisenlohr-Moul, T. and Mendle, J. (2020) 'Evolution, the menstrual cycle, and theoretical overreach', *Perspectives on Psychological Science*, 15(4), pp 1113–1130.

King, A. and Critchley, H. (2010) 'Oestrogen and progesterone regulation of inflammatory processes in the human endometrium', *The Journal of Steroid Biochemistry and Molecular Biology*, 120(2–3), pp 116–126.

King, H. (1993) 'Once upon a text: Hysteria from Hippocrates', in S.L. Gilman, H. King, R. Porter, G.S. Rousseau and E. Showalter (eds) *Hysteria beyond Freud*. Berkeley: University of California Press, pp 3–90.

King, H. (1998) *Hippocrates' Woman: Reading the Female Body in Ancient Greece*. London and New York: Routledge.

King, H. (2024) *Immaculate Forms: Uncovering the History of Women's Bodies*. London: Wellcome Collection.

King, M., Ussher, J.M. and Perz, J. (2014) 'Representations of PMS and premenstrual women in men's accounts: An analysis of online posts from PMSBuddy.com', *Women's Reproductive Health*, 1(1), pp 3–20.

King, S. (2020) 'Premenstrual syndrome (PMS) and the myth of the irrational female', in C. Bobel, I.T. Winkler, B. Fahs, K.A. Hasson, E.A. Kissling and T.-A. Roberts (eds) *The Palgrave Handbook of Critical Menstruation Studies*. Singapore: Springer, pp 287–302.

King, S. (2021) 'Menstrual leave: Good intention, poor solution', in J. Hassard and L.D. Torres (eds) *Aligning Perspectives in Gender Mainstreaming*. Cham: Springer International, pp 151–176.

King, S. (2023) 'Why menstrual leave could be bad for women', *The Conversation*. Available at: https://theconversation.com/why-menstrual-leave-could-be-bad-for-women-199568

King, S. (2024) 'Black box: The reduction and mystification of the menstrual cycle in Western school and medical education', in K. Standing, S. Parker and S. Lotter (eds) *Experiences of Menstruation from the Global South and North*. Oxford: Oxford University Press, pp 23–37.

Kleinstäuber, M., Witthoft, M. and Hiller, W. (2012) 'Cognitive-behavioral and pharmacological interventions for premenstrual syndrome or premenstrual dysphoric disorder: A meta-analysis', *Journal of Clinical Psychology in Medical Settings*, 19(3), pp 308–319.

Kleinstäuber, M., Schmelzer, K., Ditzen, B., Andersson, G., Hiller, W. and Weise, C. (2016) 'Psychosocial profile of women with premenstrual syndrome and healthy controls: A comparative study', *International Journal of Behavioral Medicine*, 23(6), pp 752–763.

Klyne, D.M., Barbe, M.F., James, G. and Hodges, P.W. (2021) 'Does the interaction between local and systemic inflammation provide a link from psychology and lifestyle to tissue health in musculoskeletal conditions?', *International Journal of Molecular Sciences*, 22(14), Article 7299.

Knaapen, L. and Weisz, G. (2008) 'The biomedical standardization of premenstrual syndrome', *Studies in History and Philosophy of Science*, 39(1), pp 120–134.

Knight, M., Bunch, K., Kenyon, S., Tuffnell, D. and Kurinczuk, J.J. (2020) 'A national population-based cohort study to investigate inequalities in maternal mortality in the United Kingdom, 2009–17', *Paediatric and Perinatal Epidemiology*, 34(4), pp 392–398.

Koeppen, B.M. and Stanton, B.A. (2017) *Berne & Levy Physiology*. 7th edn. New York: Elsevier.

Kuczmierczyk, A.R., Labrum, A.H. and Johnson, C.C. (1992) 'Perception of family and work environments in women with premenstrual syndrome', *Journal of Psychosomatic Research*, 36(8), pp 787–795.

Latham, R.G. (1848) *The Works of Thomas Sydenham*. Translated from the Latin Edition of Dr. Greenhill with a Life of the Author by R.G. Latham. London: Sydenham Soc.

Laws, S. (1990) *Issues of Blood*. Edited by J. Campling. London: Palgrave Macmillan.

Laws, S. (1992) ' "It's just the monthlies, she'll get over it": Menstrual problems and men's attitudes', *Journal of Reproductive and Infant Psychology*, 10(2), pp 117–128.

Laws, S., Hey, V. and Eagan, A. (1985) *Seeing Red: The Politics of Pre-menstrual Tension*. London: Hutchinson.

Lee, K.A. and Rittenhouse, C.A. (1992) 'Health and perimenstrual symptoms: Health outcomes for employed women who experience perimenstrual symptoms', *Women & Health*, 19(1), pp 65–78.

Letson, S. and Dancey, C.P. (1996) 'Nurses' perceptions of irritable bowel syndrome (IBS) and sufferers of IBS', *Journal of Advanced Nursing*, 23(5), pp 969–974.

Lloyd, G. (1984) *The Man of Reason; 'Male' and 'Female' in Western Philosophy*. London: Methuen & Co.

Logue, C.M. and Moos, R.H. (1986) 'Perimenstrual symptoms: Prevalence and risk factors', *Psychosomatic Medicine*, 48(6), pp 388–414.

Lopresti, A.L. (2017) 'Cognitive behaviour therapy and inflammation: A systematic review of its relationship and the potential implications for the treatment of depression', *Australian and New Zealand Journal of Psychiatry*, 51(6), pp 565–582.

Maddineshat, M., Keyvanloo, S., Lashkardoost, H., Arki, M. and Tabatabaeichehr, M. (2016) 'Effectiveness of group cognitive-behavioral therapy on symptoms of premenstrual syndrome (PMS)', *Iranian Journal of Psychiatry*, 11(1), pp 30–36.

Majd, M., Saunders, E.F.H. and Engeland, C.G. (2020) 'Inflammation and the dimensions of depression: A review', *Frontiers in Neuroendocrinology*, 56, Article 100800.

Makabe, T., Koga, K., Miyashita, M., Takeuchi, A., Sue, F., Taguchi, A., et al (2017) 'Drospirenone reduces inflammatory cytokines, vascular endothelial growth factor (VEGF) and nerve growth factor (NGF) expression in human endometriotic stromal cells', *Journal of Reproductive Immunology*, 119, pp 44–48.

Mallia, C. (2015) *The Epidemiology and Management of Premenstrual Symptoms in the Community*. PhD thesis submitted to the University of Aberdeen. Available at: https://abdn.primo.exlibrisgroup.com/discovery/delivery/44ABE_INST:44ABE_VU1/12152380480005941

Manicom, D.P. (2010) *Gender Essentialism: A Conceptual and Empirical Exploration of Notions of Maternal Essence as a Framework for Explaining Gender Difference*. PhD thesis submitted to the University of Kwazulu-Natal Available at: https://researchspace.ukzn.ac.za/handle/10413/7524

Marjoribanks, J., Ayeleke, R.O., Farquhar, C. and Proctor, M. (2015) 'Nonsteroidal anti-inflammatory drugs for dysmenorrhoea', *Cochrane Database of Systematic Reviews*, 7, Article CD001751.

Martin, E. (1987) *The Woman in the Body: A Cultural Analysis of Reproduction*. Milton Keynes: Open University Press.

Marván, M. and Escobedo, C. (1999) 'Premenstrual symptomatology: Role of prior knowledge about premenstrual syndrome', *Psychosomatic Medicine*, 61(2), pp 163–167.

Maybin, J.A. and Critchley, H.O.D. (2015) 'Menstrual physiology: Implications for endometrial pathology and beyond', *Human Reproduction Update*, 21(6), pp 748–761.

Maybin, J.A., Critchley, H.O.D. and Jabbour, H.N. (2011) 'Inflammatory pathways in endometrial disorders', *Molecular and Cellular Endocrinology*, 335(1), pp 42–51.

McFarlane, J. and Williams, T. (1994) 'Placing premenstrual syndrome in perspective', *Psychology of Women Quarterly*, 18(3), pp 339–373.

McFarlane, J., Martin, C. and Williams, T. (1988) 'Mood fluctuations: Women versus men and menstrual versus other cycles', *Psychology of Women Quarterly*, 12(2), pp 201–223.

McGarvey, A., Jochum, V., Davies, J., Dobbs, J. and Hornung, L. (2020) *Time Well Spent: A National Survey on the Volunteering Experience*. Available at: https://www.ncvo.org.uk/policy-and-research/volunteering-policy/research/time-well-spent

McHugh, M. and Chrisler, J. (2015) *The Wrong Prescription for Women: How Medicine and Media Create a 'Need' for Treatments, Drugs, and Surgery*. New York: Praeger.

Mende-Siedlecki, P., Qu-Lee, J., Backer, R. and Van Bavel, J.J. (2019) 'Perceptual contributions to racial bias in pain recognition', *Journal of Experimental Psychology: General*, 148(5), pp 863–889.

Micale, M.S. (2019) *Approaching Hysteria*. 2nd edn. Princeton: Princeton University Press.

Miccio-Fonseca, L.C., Jones, J.E. and Futterman, L.A. (1990) 'Sexual trauma and the premenstrual syndrome', *Journal of Sex Education and Therapy*, 16(4), pp 270–278.

Miller, G., Tybur, J.M. and Jordan, B.D. (2007) 'Ovulatory cycle effects on tip earnings by lap dancers: Economic evidence for human estrus?', *Evolution and Human Behavior*, 28(6), pp 375–381.

Miller, S. (2022) 'Women open up about "torturous pain" after nurse at infertility clinic steals pain meds', *NBC*, 24 May. Available at: https://www.nbcconnecticut.com/investigations/women-open-up-about-tortur ous-pain-after-nurse-at-infertility-clinic-steals-pain-meds/2792701/

Mirin, A.A. (2021) 'Gender disparity in the funding of diseases by the U.S. National Institutes of Health', *Journal of Women's Health*, 30(7), pp 956–963.

Modugno, F., Ness, R.B., Chen, C. and Weiss, N.S. (2005) 'Inflammation and endometrial cancer: A hypothesis', *Cancer Epidemiology Biomarkers and Prevention*, 14(12), pp 2840–2847.

Mohammadi, M.M., Nayeri, N.D., Mashhadi, M. and Varaei, S. (2022) 'Effect of omega-3 fatty acids on premenstrual syndrome: A systematic review and meta-analysis', *Journal of Obstetrics and Gynaecology Research*, 48(6), pp 1293–1305.

Mukwende, M., Tamonv, P. and Turner, M. (2020) *Mind the Gap: A Handbook of Clinical Signs in Black and Brown Skin*. 1st edn. London: St George's University. Available at: https://www.blackandbrownskin.co.uk/ mindthegap

Muljat, A.M., Lustyk, M.K.B. and Miller, A. (2007) 'Stress moderates the effects of premenstrual symptomatology on body image reports in women', *Annals of Behavioral Medicine*, 33, pp 157–158.

Myers, B.E.I. (2014) *'Drapetomania' Rebellion, Defiance and Free Black Insanity in the Antebellum United States*. PhD thesis submitted to the University of California. Available at: https://www.proquest.com/dissertations-the ses/drapetomania-rebellion-defiance-free-black/docview/1648436283/ se-2?accountid=11862

NICE (2023) *Anaemia – Iron Deficiency*. Available at: https://cks.nice.org. uk/topics/anaemia-iron-deficiency/

Nowosielski, K., Drosdzol, A., Skrzypulec, V. and Plinta, R. (2010) 'Sexual satisfaction in females with premenstrual symptoms', *The Journal of Sexual Medicine*, 7(11), pp 3589–3597.

O'Brien, P.M.S. and Ismail, K.M.K. (2007) 'History of the premenstrual disorders', in P.M.S. O'Brien, A. Rapkin and P.J. Schmidt (eds) *The Premenstrual Syndromes: PMS and PMDD*. London: CRC Press, pp 1–8.

O'Flynn, N. and Britten, N. (2000) 'Menorrhagia in general practice: Disease or illness', *Social Science & Medicine*, 50(5), pp 651–661.

Ohde, S., Tokuda, Y., Takahashi, O., Yanai, H., Hinohara, S. and Fukui, T. (2008) 'Dysmenorrhea among Japanese women', *International Journal of Gynecology & Obstetrics*, 100(1), pp 13–17.

Ojeda-Ojeda, M., Murri, M., Insenser, M. and Escobar-Morreale, H.F. (2013) 'Mediators of low-grade chronic inflammation in polycystic ovary syndrome (PCOS)', *Current Pharmaceutical Design*, 19(32), pp 5775–5791.

ONS (2020) *Overview of the UK Population: November 2018*. London: ONS. Available at: https://www.ons.gov.uk/peoplepopulationandcommunity/ populationandmigration/populationestimates/articles/overviewoftheuk population/november2018

Orhan, C., Van Looveren, E., Cagnie, B., Mukhtar, N.B., Lenoir, D. and Meeus, M. (2018) 'Are pain beliefs, cognitions, and behaviors influenced by race, ethnicity, and culture in patients with chronic musculoskeletal pain: A systematic review', *Pain Physician*, 21(6), pp 541–558.

Oudshoorn, N. (2003) *Beyond the Natural Body: An Archaeology of Sex Hormones*. London and New York: Routledge.

Palacios-Ceña, D., Neira-Martín, B., Silva-Hernández, L., Mayo-Canalejo, D., Florencio, L.L., Fernández-de-Las-Peñas, C., et al (2017) 'Living with chronic migraine: A qualitative study on female patients' perspectives from a specialised headache clinic in Spain', *BMJ Open*, 7(8), Article e017851.

Palinkas, L.A., Horwitz, S.M., Green, C.A., Wisdom, J.P., Duan, N. and Hoagwood, K. (2015) 'Purposeful sampling for qualitative data collection and analysis in mixed method implementation research', *Administration and Policy in Mental Health and Mental Health Services Research*, 42(5), pp 533–544.

Parboteeah, K.P., Cullen, J.B. and Lim, L. (2004) 'Formal volunteering: A cross-national test', *Journal of World Business*, 39(4), pp 431–441.

Parlee, M.B. (1987) 'Media treatment of premenstrual syndrome', in B.E. Ginsburg and B.F. Carter (eds) *Premenstrual Syndrome: Ethical and Legal Implications in a Biomedical Perspective*. Boston: Springer US, pp 189–205.

Pateman, C. (1988) *The Sexual Contract*. Stanford: Stanford University Press

Payne, J.L. and Maguire, J. (2019) 'Pathophysiological mechanisms implicated in postpartum depression', *Frontiers in Neuroendocrinology*, 52, pp 165–180.

Percy, L., Mansour, D. and Fraser, I. (2017) 'Iron deficiency and iron deficiency anaemia in women', *Best Practice & Research Clinical Obstetrics & Gynaecology*, 40, pp 55–67.

Perkonigg, A., Yonkers, K.A., Pfister, H., Lieb, R. and Wittchen, H.-U. (2004) 'Risk factors for premenstrual dysphoric disorder in a community sample of young women: The role of traumatic events and posttraumatic stress disorder', *Journal of Clinical Psychiatry*, 65, pp 1314–1322.

Petta, C.A., Osis, M.J.D., de Pádua, K.S., Bahamondes, L. and Makuch, M.Y. (2010) 'Premenstrual syndrome as reported by Brazilian women', *International Journal of Gynecology & Obstetrics*, 108(1), pp 40–43.

Pilver, C.E., Kasl, S., Desai, R. and Levy, B.R. (2011) 'Exposure to American culture is associated with premenstrual dysphoric disorder among ethnic minority women', *Journal of Affective Disorders*, 130(1–2), pp 334–341.

Pinho, M. and Gaunt, R. (2024) 'Biological essentialism, gender ideologies, and the division of housework and childcare: Comparing male carer/female breadwinner and traditional families', *The Journal of Social Psychology*, 164(1), pp 59–75.

Plant, T.M. and Zeleznik, A.J. (2015) *Knobil and Neill's Physiology of Reproduction: Two-Volume Set*. Cham: Elsevier.

Potter, J., Sari, Z. and Lindblad, A.J. (2021) 'NSAIDs for heavy menstrual bleeding', *Canadian Family Physician*, 67(8), pp 598–599.

Putnam Jacobi, M. (1876) *The Question of Rest for Women during Menstruation: The Boylston Prize Essay of Harvard University for 1876*. Cambridge, MA: Harvard University Press. Available at: https://digirepo.nlm.nih.gov/ext/kirtasbse/67041010R/PDF/67041010R.pdf

Quintana-Zinn, F.A., Whitcomb, B.W., Ronnenberg, A.G., Bigelow, C., Houghton, S.C. and Bertone-Johnson, E.R. (2017) 'Premenstrual symptom patterns and behavioral risk factors in young women: A cross-sectional study', *Journal of Women's Health*, 26(10), pp 1099–1105.

Quirke, S. (2002) *Manuscript for the Health of Mother and Child*. Translated by The Kahun Gynaecological Papyrus. Available at: http://www.ucl.ac.uk/museums-static/digitalegypt/med/birthpapyrus.html

Rana, A. and Musto, A.E. (2018) 'The role of inflammation in the development of epilepsy', *Journal of Neuroinflammation*, 15(1), Article 144.

RCOG (2016) 'Management of premenstrual syndrome: Green-top guideline no. 48', *BJOG: An International Journal of Obstetrics & Gynaecology*, 124(3), pp 73–105.

Read, J.R., Perz, J. and Ussher, J.M. (2014) 'Ways of coping with premenstrual change: Development and validation of a premenstrual coping measure', *BMC Women's Health*, 14(1).

Regan, L. and Rai, R. (2000) 'Epidemiology and the medical causes of miscarriage', *Best Practice & Research Clinical Obstetrics & Gynaecology*, 14(5), pp 839–854.

Renna, M.E., O'Toole, M.S., Spaeth, P.E., Lekander, M. and Mennin, D.S. (2018) 'The association between anxiety, traumatic stress, and obsessive–compulsive disorders and chronic inflammation: A systematic review and meta-analysis', *Depression and Anxiety*, 35(11), pp 1081–1094.

Rier, S.E. and Yeaman, G.R. (2008) 'Immune aspects of endometriosis: Relevance of the uterine mucosal immune system', *Seminars in Reproductive Endocrinology*, 15(3), pp 209–220.

Rittenhouse, C.A. (1991) 'The emergence of premenstrual syndrome as a social problem', *Social Problems*, 38(3), pp 412–425.

Roberts, C. (2007) *Messengers of Sex*. Cambridge: Cambridge University Press.

Roberts, I. and Jones, C.P. (2023) 'Structural racism and iron deficiency anaemia', *The Lancet*, 402(10405), pp 834–835.

Robillard, P.Y., Dekker, G.A. and Hulsey, T.C. (2002) 'Evolutionary adaptations to pre-eclampsia/eclampsia in humans: Low fecundability rate, loss of oestrus, prohibitions of incest and systematic polyandry', *American Journal of Reproductive Immunology*, 47(2), pp 104–111.

Robillard, P.-Y., Dekker, G., Chaouat, G., Elliot, M.G. and Scioscia, M. (2019) 'High incidence of early onset preeclampsia is probably the rule and not the exception worldwide. 20th anniversary of the reunion workshop. A summary', *Journal of Reproductive Immunology*, 133, pp 30–36.

Rodin, M. (1992) 'The social construction of premenstrual syndrome', *Social Science & Medicine*, 35(1), pp 49–56.

Romans, S., Clarkson, R., Einstein, G., Petrovic, M. and Stewart, D. (2012) 'Mood and the menstrual cycle: A review of prospective data studies', *Gender Medicine*, 9(5), pp 361–384.

Roth, W.D., van Stee, E.G. and Regla-Vargas, A. (2023) 'Conceptualizations of race: Essentialism and constructivism', *Annual Review of Sociology*, 49(1), pp 39–58.

Rubinow, D. and Schmidt, P. (1995) 'The neuroendocrinology of menstrual cycle mood disorders', *Annals of the New York Academy of Sciences*, 771(1), pp 648–659.

Rubinow, D. and Schmidt, P. (2006) 'Gonadal steroid regulation of mood: The lessons of premenstrual syndrome', *Frontiers in Neuroendocrinology*, 27(2), pp 210–216.

Rubinow, D.R., Hoban, M.C., Grover, G.N., Galloway, D.S., Roy-Byrne, P., Andersen, R., et al (1988) 'Changes in plasma hormones across the menstrual cycle in patients with menstrually related mood disorder and in control subjects', *American Journal of Obstetrics and Gynecology*, 158(1), pp 5–11.

Ruble, D.N. (1977) 'Premenstrual symptoms: A reinterpretation', *Science*, 197(4300), pp 291–292.

Ryser, R. and Feinauer, L.L. (1992) 'Premenstrual syndrome and the marital relationship', *The American Journal of Family Therapy*, 20(2), pp 179–190.

Saguy, T., Reifen-Tagar, M. and Joel, D. (2021) 'The gender-binary cycle: The perpetual relations between a biological-essentialist view of gender, gender ideology, and gender-labelling and sorting', *Philosophical Transactions of the Royal Society B: Biological Sciences*, 376(1822), Article 20200141.

Salamonsen, L. (2021) 'Menstrual fluid factors mediate endometrial repair', *Frontiers in Reproductive Health*, 3, Article 779979.

Salamonsen, L. and Woolley, D.E. (1999) 'Menstruation: Induction by matrix metalloproteinases and inflammatory cells', *Journal of Reproductive Immunology*, 44(1–2), pp 1–27.

Santer, M., Wyke, S. and Warner, P. (2008) 'Women's management of menstrual symptoms: Findings from a postal survey and qualitative interviews', *Social Science & Medicine*, 66(2), pp 276–288.

Scambler, G. and Scambler, A. (1993) *Menstrual Disorders*. 1st edn. London and New York: Routledge.

Schaffir, J., Worly, B.L. and Gur, T.L. (2016) 'Combined hormonal contraception and its effects on mood: A critical review', *European Journal of Contraception and Reproductive Health Care*, 21(5), pp 347–355.

Schmalenberger, K.M., Tauseef, H.A., Barone, J.C., Owens, S.A., Lieberman, L., Jarczok, M.N., et al (2021) 'How to study the menstrual cycle: Practical tools and recommendations', *Psychoneuroendocrinology*, 123, Article 104895.

Schmelzer, K., Ditzen, B., Weise, C., Andersson, G., Hiller, W. and Kleinstäuber, M. (2015) 'Clinical profiles of premenstrual experiences among women having premenstrual syndrome (PMS): Affective changes predominate and relate to social and occupational functioning', *Health Care for Women International*, 36(10), pp 1104–1123.

Schmidt, J., Weijdegård, B., Mikkelsen, A.L., Lindenberg, S., Nilsson, L. and Brännström, M. (2014) 'Differential expression of inflammation-related genes in the ovarian stroma and granulosa cells of PCOS women', *Molecular Human Reproduction*, 20(1), pp 49–58.

Schmidt, P.J., Nieman, L.K., Danaceau, M.A., Adams, L.F. and Rubinow, D.R. (1998) 'Differential behavioral effects of gonadal steroids in women with and in those without premenstrual syndrome', *New England Journal of Medicine*, 338(4), pp 209–216.

Segebladh, B., Borgström, A., Odlind, V., Bixo, M. and Sundström-Poromaa, I. (2009) 'Prevalence of psychiatric disorders and premenstrual dysphoric symptoms in patients with experience of adverse mood during treatment with combined oral contraceptives', *Contraception*, 79(1), pp 50–55.

Sharma, S., Reimer-Kirkham, S. and Cochrane, M. (2009) 'Practicing the awareness of embodiment in qualitative health research: Methodological reflections', *Qualitative Health Research*, 19(11), pp 1642–1650.

Sharma, V., Mazmanian, D. and Eccles, H. (2022) 'Relationship of premenstrual dysphoric disorder with bipolar disorder: A systematic review', *The Journal of Clinical Psychiatry*, 83(6), Article 43549.

Sharman, L.S., Dingle, G.A., Baker, M., Fischer, A., Gračanin, A., Kardum, I., et al (2019) 'The relationship of gender roles and beliefs to crying in an international sample', *Frontiers in Psychology*, 10, Article 2288.

Shattuck, E.C. and Muehlenbein, M.P. (2015) 'Human sickness behavior: Ultimate and proximate explanations', *American Journal of Physical Anthropology*, 157(1), pp 1–18.

Shorakae, S., Ranasinha, S., Abell, S., Lambert, G., Lambert, E., de Courten, B., et al (2018) 'Inter-related effects of insulin resistance, hyperandrogenism, sympathetic dysfunction and chronic inflammation in PCOS', *Clinical Endocrinology*, 89(5), pp 628–633.

Showalter, E. (1993) 'Hysteria, feminism, and gender', in S.L. Gilman (ed) *Hysteria beyond Freud*. Berkeley: University of California Press, pp 286–344.

Simmons, R.G. and Jennings, V. (2020) 'Fertility awareness-based methods of family planning', *Best Practice & Research Clinical Obstetrics & Gynaecology*, 66, pp 68–82.

Simon, C., Everitt, H., van Dorp, F. and Burkes, M. (2014) *Oxford Handbook of General Practice*. Oxford: Oxford University Press.

Sims-Schouten, W. and Riley, S. (2014) 'Employing a form of critical realist discourse analysis for identity research: An example from women's talk of motherhood, childcare, and employment', in P.K. Edwards, J. O'Mahoney and S. Vincent (eds) *Studying Organizations Using Critical Realism: A Practical Guide*. Oxford: Oxford University Press, pp 46–65.

Sims-Schouten, W., Riley, S.C.E. and Willig, C. (2007) 'Critical realism in discourse analysis', *Theory & Psychology*, 17(1), pp 101–124.

Sinha, M., Patel, A.H., Naik, S. and Jadeja, J.M. (2013) 'Effect of anemia on premenstrual syndrome in adolescent girls', *International Journal of Basic and Applied Physiology*, 2(1), pp 104–108.

Smorgick, N., Marsh, C.A., As-Sanie, S., Smith, Y.R. and Quint, E.H. (2013) 'Prevalence of pain syndromes, mood conditions, and asthma in adolescents and young women with endometriosis', *Journal of Pediatric and Adolescent Gynecology*, 26(3), pp 171–175.

Southam, A.L. and Gonzaga, F.P. (1965) 'Systemic changes during the menstrual cycle', *American Journal of Obstetrics and Gynecology*, 91(1), pp 142–165.

Stach, K., Stach, W. and Augoff, K. (2021) 'Vitamin B6 in health and disease', *Nutrients*, 13(9), Article 3229.

Stepan, N.L. (1986) 'Race and gender: The role of analogy in science', *Isis*, 77(2), pp 261–277.

Sveinsdóttir, H. (1998) 'Prospective assessment of menstrual and premenstrual experiences of Icelandic women', *Health Care for Women International*, 19(1), pp 71–82.

Sveinsdóttir, H. and Bäckström, T. (2000) 'Menstrual cycle symptom variation in a community sample of women using and not using oral contraceptives', *Acta Obstetricia et Gynecologica Scandinavica*, 79(9), pp 757–764.

Szasz, T.S. (1960) 'The myth of mental illness', *American Psychologist*, 15(2), pp 113–118.

Tan, D.A., Haththotuwa, R. and Fraser, I.S. (2017) 'Cultural aspects and mythologies surrounding menstruation and abnormal uterine bleeding', *Best Practice & Research Clinical Obstetrics & Gynaecology*, 40, pp 121–133.

Tang, P. and Wang, J.M. (2018) 'Chemokines: The past, the present and the future', *Cellular & Molecular Immunology*, 15(4), pp 295–298.

Tasca, C., Rapetti, M., Carta, M.G. and Fadda, B. (2012) 'Women and hysteria in the history of mental health', *Clinical Practice & Epidemiology in Mental Health*, 8(1), pp 110–119.

Tax Policy Associates (2022) *How the Abolition of the 'Tampon Tax' Benefited Retailers, Not Women.* Available at: https://taxpolicy.org.uk/assets/tampon_tax_report.pdf

Taylor, D. (2006) 'From "it's all in your head" to "taking back the month": Premenstrual syndrome (PMS) research and the contributions of the society for menstrual cycle research', *Sex Roles*, 54(5–6), pp 377–391.

Taylor, H.S., Adamson, G.D., Diamond, M.P., Goldstein, S.R., Horne, A.W., Missmer, S.A., et al (2018) 'An evidence-based approach to assessing surgical versus clinical diagnosis of symptomatic endometriosis', *International Journal of Gynaecology and Obstetrics*, 142, pp 131–142.

Ternhag, A., Asikainen, T. and Giesecke, J. (2005) 'Size matters: Patient organisations exaggerate prevalence numbers', *European Journal of Epidemiology*, 20(8), pp 653–655.

Thomas, P. and Bracken, P. (2004) 'Critical psychiatry in practice', *Advances in Psychiatric Treatment*, 10(5), pp 361–370.

Thong, I.S.K., Tan, G., Lee, T.Y.C. and Jensen, M.P. (2017) 'A comparison of pain beliefs and coping strategies and their association with chronic pain adjustment between Singapore and United States', *Pain Medicine (United States)*, 18(9), pp 1668–1678.

Tingle, C. and Vora, S. (2018) *Break the Barriers: Girls' Experiences of Menstruation in the UK.* London: Plan International UK.

Tourangeau, R. (1999) 'Remembering what happened: Memory errors and survey reports', in A.A. Stone, J.S. Turkkan, C.A. Bachrach, J.B. Jobe, H.S. Kurtzman and V.S. Cain (eds) *The Science of Self-report.* Oxford: Psychology Press, pp 41–60.

Trimble, M. and Reynolds, E.H. (2016) 'A brief history of hysteria', in M. Hallett, J. Stone and A. Carson (eds) *Handbook of Clinical Neurology.* Cham: Elsevier, pp 3–10.

Ussher, J.M. (1989) *The Psychology of the Female Body.* London and New York: Routledge.

Ussher, J.M. (2003) 'The ongoing silencing of women in families: An analysis and rethinking of premenstrual syndrome and therapy', *Journal of Family Therapy*, 25(4), pp 388–405.

Ussher, J.M. (2004) 'Premenstrual syndrome and self-policing: Ruptures in self-silencing leading to increased self-surveillance and blaming of the body', *Social Theory and Health*, 2(3), pp 254–272.

Ussher, J.M (2005) *Managing the Monstrous Feminine: Regulating the Reproductive Body.* London and New York: Routledge.

Ussher, J.M. (2011) *The Madness of Women: Myth and Experience*. London and New York: Routledge.

Ussher, J.M. and Perz, J. (2013a) 'PMS as a gendered illness linked to the construction and relational experience of hetero-femininity', *Sex Roles*, 68(1–2), pp 132–150.

Ussher, J.M. and Perz, J. (2013b) 'PMS as a process of negotiation: Women's experience and management of premenstrual distress', *Psychology & Health*, 28(8), pp 909–927.

Ussher, J.M. and Perz, J. (2017) 'Evaluation of the relative efficacy of a couple cognitive-behaviour therapy (CBT) for Premenstrual Disorders (PMDs), in comparison to one-to-one CBT and a wait list control: A randomized controlled trial', *PLOS ONE*, 12(4), Article e0175068.

Ussher, J.M. and Perz, J. (2020a) ' "I feel fat and ugly and hate myself": Self-objectification through negative constructions of premenstrual embodiment', *Feminism & Psychology*, 30(2), pp 185–205.

Ussher, J.M. and Perz, J. (2020b) 'Resisting the mantle of the monstrous feminine: Women's construction and experience of premenstrual embodiment', in C. Bobel, I.T. Winkler, B. Fahs, K.A. Hasson, E.A. Kissling and T.-A. Roberts (eds) *The Palgrave Handbook of Critical Menstruation Studies*. New York: Palgrave Macmillan, pp 215–231.

Ussher, J.M., Perz, J. and Mooney-Somers, J. (2007) 'The experience and positioning of affect in the context of intersubjectivity: The case of premenstrual syndrome', *International Journal of Critical Psychology*, 21, pp 144–165.

Ussher, J.M., Rhyder-Obid, M., Perz, J., Rae, M., Wong, T.W.K. and Newman, P. (2012) 'Purity, privacy and procreation: Constructions and experiences of sexual and reproductive health in Assyrian and Karen women living in Australia', *Sexuality & Culture*, 16(4), pp 467–485.

Ussher, J.M., Perz, J., Metusela, C., Hawkey, A.J., Morrow, M., Narchal, R., et al (2017) 'Negotiating discourses of shame, secrecy, and silence: Migrant and refugee women's experiences of sexual embodiment', *Archives of Sexual Behavior*, 46(7), pp 1901–1921.

Ussher, J.M, Chrisler, J. and Perz, J. (2019) *Routledge International Handbook of Women's Sexual and Reproductive Health*. London and New York: Routledge.

van Iersel, K.C., Kiesner, J., Pastore, M. and Scholte, R.H.J. (2016) 'The impact of menstrual cycle-related physical symptoms on daily activities and psychological wellness among adolescent girls', *Journal of Adolescence*, 49(1), pp 81–90.

Van Tilburg, M.A.L., Becht, M.C. and Vingerhoets, A.J.J.M. (2003) 'Self-reported crying during the menstrual cycle: Sign of discomfort and emotional turmoil or erroneous beliefs?', *Journal of Psychosomatic Obstetrics and Gynecology*, 24(4), pp 247–255.

Veith, I. (1965) *Hysteria: The History of a Disease*. Chicago: University of Chicago Press.

Vingerhoets, A.J.J.M., Rottenberg, J., Cevaal, A. and Nelson, J.K. (2007) 'Is there a relationship between depression and crying? A review', *Acta Psychiatrica Scandinavica*, 115(5), pp 340–351.

Walker, A. (1995a) 'Theory and methodology in premenstrual syndrome research', *Social Science and Medicine*, 41(6), pp 793–800.

Walker, A.E. (1995b) 'Premenstrual syndrome', *International Journal of Gynecology & Obstetrics*, 50(1), pp 80–84.

Walker, A.E. (1997) *The Menstrual Cycle*. London and New York: Routledge.

Walley-Jean, J.C. (2009) 'Debunking the myth of the "angry black woman": An exploration of anger in young African American women', *Women, Gender + Families*, 3(2), pp 68–86.

Wandner, L.D., Scipio, C.D., Hirsh, A.T., Torres, C.A. and Robinson, M.E. (2012) 'The perception of pain in others: How gender, race, and age influence pain expectations', *Journal of Pain*, 13(3), pp 220–227.

Warner, P. and Bancroft, J. (1990) 'Factors related to self-reporting of the pre-menstrual syndrome', *British Journal of Psychiatry*, 157(1), pp 249–260.

Warner, P., Bancroft, J., Dixson, A. and Hampson, M. (1991) 'The relationship between perimenstrual depressive mood and depressive illness', *Journal of Affective Disorders*, 23(1), pp 9–23.

Wassef, A., Nguyen, Q.D. and St-André, M. (2019) 'Anaemia and depletion of iron stores as risk factors for postpartum depression: A literature review', *Journal of Psychosomatic Obstetrics and Gynaecology*, 40(1), pp 19–28.

Weisse, C.S., Sorum, P.C., Sanders, K.N. and Syat, B.L. (2001) 'Do gender and race affect decisions about pain management?', *Journal of General Internal Medicine*, 16(4), pp 211–217.

Weiss-Wolf, J. (2017) *Periods Gone Public: Taking a Stand for Menstrual Equity*. New York: Arcade.

Weisz, G. and Knaapen, L. (2009) 'Diagnosing and treating premenstrual syndrome in five western nations', *Social Science & Medicine*, 68(8), pp 1498–1505.

Westwood, S., Fannin, M., Ali, F., Thigpen, J., Tatro, R., Hernandez, A., et al (2023) 'Disparities in women with endometriosis regarding access to care, diagnosis, treatment, and management in the United States: A scoping review', *Cureus*, 15(5).

Whitaker, L.H.R., Arulkumaran, S., Ledger, W., Denny, L. and Doumouchtsis, S. (eds) (2020) *Oxford Textbook of Obstetrics and Gynaecology*. 1st edn. Oxford: Oxford University Press.

White, B., Harrison, J.R. and Mehlmann, L. (2018) *Endocrine and Reproductive Physiology*. 4th edn. Cham: Elsevier.

White, C.P., Hitchcock, C.L., Vigna, Y.M. and Prior, J.C. (2011) 'Fluid retention over the menstrual cycle: 1-year data from the prospective ovulation cohort', *Obstetrics and Gynecology International*, 2011, Article 138451.

WHO (2023) *Maternal Mortality Factsheet*, *World Health Organisation*. Available at: https://www.who.int/news-room/fact-sheets/detail/maternal-mortality

Wiggins, S. (2017) *Discursive Psychology: Theory, Method and Applications*. 1st edn. London: SAGE.

Wilkinson, S. and Kitzinger, C. (1994) *Women and Health: Feminist Perspectives*. Oxford: Taylor & Francis.

Williams, R.L., Romney, C., Kano, M., Wright, R., Skipper, B., Getrich, C.M., et al (2015) 'Racial, gender, and socioeconomic status bias in senior medical student clinical decision-making: A national survey', *Journal of General Internal Medicine*, 30(6), pp 758–767.

Williams, S.J., Birke, L. and Bendelow, G.A. (2003) *Debating Biology: Sociological Reflections on Health, Medicine and Society*. Oxford: Routledge.

Wilson, E.A. (2005) 'Gut feminism', *Differences*, 15(3), pp 66–94.

Woods, N.F., Taylor, D., Mitchell, E.S. and Lentz, M.J. (1992) 'Perimenstrual symptoms and health-seeking behavior', *Western Journal of Nursing Research*, 14(4), pp 418–443.

Xu, X., Jiang, W., Chen, L., Xu, Z., Zhang, Q., Zhu, M., et al (2021) 'Evaluation of the safety and efficacy of using human menstrual blood-derived mesenchymal stromal cells in treating severe and critically ill COVID-19 patients: An exploratory clinical trial', *Clinical and Translational Medicine*, 11(2), Article e297.

Yu, L., Wang, L. and Chen, S. (2009) 'Toll-like receptors, inflammation and tumor in the human female reproductive tract', *American Journal of Reproductive Immunology*, 62(1), pp 1–8.

Yu, M., Zhu, X., Li, J., Oakley, D. and Reame, N.E. (1996) 'Perimenstrual symptoms among Chinese women in an urban area of China', *Health Care for Women International*, 17(2), pp 161–172.

Zeitoun, T., Noudeh, N.D., Garcia-Bailo, B. and El-Sohemy, A. (2021) 'Genetics of iron metabolism and premenstrual symptoms: A Mendelian randomization study', *Journal of Nutrition*, 151(7), pp 1747–1754.

Zendehdel, M. and Elyasi, F. (2018) 'Biopsychosocial etiology of premenstrual syndrome: A narrative review', *Journal of Family Medicine and Primary Care*, 7(2), pp 346–356.

Zhou, H.-G., Yang, Z.-W. and Group, S. (2010) 'Prevalence of dysmenorrhea in female students in a Chinese university: A prospective study', *Health*, 2(4), pp 311–314.

Zukerstein, J. (2015) 'Discursive mechanisms of legitimization: A framework for analysis', *European Scientific Journal*, 1, pp 292–296.

Index

References to figures appear in *italic* type; those in **bold** type refer to tables.

A

abdominal pain 95, 99, **115**
  consulting a doctor over 90, **92**
  minimisation of 90, 93–95, **94**, 97, 101
  prioritising of mood changes
    over 91, 103
  as secondary dysmenorrhea 97
abortion, natural 14, 19, 20,
  164, 182n8ch1
action, call to 160–164
  clinicians and healthcare
    professionals 161–163
  moving forward in women's
    health 160, 164
  research scientists 160–161
  wider society 163–164
'all in the mind' gender myth
  influence on participant group
    discourses 180, 181
  premenstrual changes as 67–73, 79,
    80, 81
    biomedical perspectives and PMS
      stereotype 71–73
    Black and ethnic minorities 70
    critical perspectives and PMS
      stereotype 71
    disbelief in patient experiences 68–70,
      69, 79, 81
American College of Obstetrics and
  Gynaecology (ACOG) 138
American Psychiatric Association 35, **36**,
  37, 56, **83**
anaemia, iron-deficiency 22–23, 50, 90,
  132–133, **132**, 159
  treating 163
Ancient Greeks 27, 29
anti-inflammatory medications 22, 99, 135

B

Bancroft, J. 50
biomedical experts
  alternative labelling of premenstrual
    changes 99, **100**
  comparisons of description of PMS
    symptoms in population data vs
    145–146, **147**
  descriptions of PMS 64–66, **67**, 78
  difficulty in distinguishing between
    healthy and debilitating premenstrual
    symptoms 130–131, 142

  discourse on why premenstrual symptoms
    occur 104–106
  uptake of discourse by others
    107–108, 120
  discursive 'sex difference' within
    group 109–110
  emergence of biomedical PMS 26,
    32–36, 40, 186n48
  why this matters 42–43
  equating menstrual cycle with
    'fluctuating hormones' only 131–133,
    132, *134*, 135, 152–153
  estimating number of PMS
    symptoms 116–117
  estimating prevalence of PMS 86, 118,
    119–120, *119*, 121
  gender myths influencing discourse 150,
    153, 180
  gendered symptoms and treatments 110,
    111, 112–113
  and influence of PMS stereotype on
    perspectives 71–73
  legitimising rhetoric 120, 139, 156
  lists of most common premenstrual
    symptoms **67**, 115–116, **115**
  maintaining 'hormonal' discourse despite
    contradictory data 133–136, 142
  medicalisation of premenstrual
    changes 85–87, 87–89, **88**,
    100–101, 101
  minimisation of debilitating menstrual
    symptoms 90–91, **94**
  overemphasis of some symptoms
    87–88, **88**
  positioning of PMDD 74–75, 78
  psychiatry vs gynaecology 136–140, 142
  unnecessary separation of critical and 157
  views on current definition of
    PMS 114–116, 121
biopsychosocial factors in Premenstrual
  Syndrome 48–51, 62
  biological factors 50–51
  Critical Realist approach 51
  PMS as embodied interpersonal
    stress 49–50
  PMS as priming 48–49
  possible reasons for omission from
    biomedical guidelines 50–51, 62
  research 160
black box *see* 'female body as mysterious'
  myth informing 'black box' discourse

'bloating' **88**, 93, **94**, 99, **115**
  'bowel changes' and 112
  patients' views on 111–112
body image, negative 49, 111–112,
  121, 146

C

capitalism, advent of 30–31
Chrisler, Joan 17, 39, 70
clinical practice, why this matters to
  black box 144
  the curse 123
  from hysterical to hormonal 42–43
  mind over matter 81
  reduction and mystification of menstrual
    cycle 24
  snatch-22 102–103
  what counts as premenstrual
    symptoms 63
clinicians
  call to action 161–163
  interdisciplinary difficulties between
    'feminists' and 140–141
  patients' experiences of consulting
    69–70, 90, 91–92, **92**, 128–130, 141
  poor training in menstrual
    physiology 11–13, *12*, 142, 156–157,
    158–159
Clinton, Hillary *41*
coding tree, discourse 176–179
colonial biases 5
colonisation, hormones in justification for 34
contraceptive medication 20
craniometry 31
crime and 'PMS defence' 34, 37
critical experts
  comparisons of descriptions of PMS
    symptoms in population data vs
    145–146, **147**
  descriptions of PMS 66, **67**, 78–79
  difficulty in distinguishing between
    healthy and debilitating premenstrual
    symptoms 130–131
  emergence of critical PMS 36–42
  estimating number of PMS
    symptoms 117
  estimating prevalence of PMS 118
  gender myths influencing discourse 150,
    153, 181
  and influence of PMS stereotype on
    perspectives 71
  list of most common premenstrual
    symptoms **67**, 115–116, **115**
  medicalisation of premenstrual
    symptoms 83–84, 87–89, **88**, 101
  minimisation of debilitating menstrual
    symptoms 92–93, **94**
  not invited to meetings on formal PMS
    definition 140–141

perspectives on PMDD 76–77
positivism vs social constructionism
  140–141, 142–143
unnecessary separation of biomedical
  and 135
use of terms relating to healthy
  premenstrual physiology 131, 132, **132**
on why premenstrual symptoms
  occur 107, 120
Critical Realist Discourse Analysis
  (CRDA) 55–61, 145, 158
  excerpts v. quotes and their labelling 61
  step 1: Discursive Psychology
    analysis 56
  step 2: (Rhetorical) Discourse
    Analysis 56–58, 176–179
  step 3: Extra-discursive analysis 58–59,
    59, 136
  step 4: Data triangulation 59–61, **60**
cultural norms and beliefs in perceptions of
  Premenstrual Syndrome 39, 49
the curse *see* 'femininity as debility' myth
  informing discourse of 'the curse'

D

Dalton, Katharina 34, 116, 117
data collection and analysis *see*
  study comparing discourses on
  Premenstrual Syndrome
data triangulation 59–61, **60**
Dennerstein, Lorraine **60**, 61, **67**, **88**,
  94, **147**
Descartes, R. 30
Discourse Analysis (DA) *see* Critical Realist
  Discourse Analysis (CRDA)
discourse coding tree 176–179
discursive device notation 55, 174–175
Discursive Psychology analysis 56
doctors
  call to action 161–163
  interdisciplinary difficulties between
    'feminists' and 140–141
  patients' experiences of consulting 69–70,
    90, 91–92, **92**, 128–130, 141
  poor training in menstrual
    physiology 11–13, *12*, 142, 156–157,
    158–159
drapetomania 31
DSM V diagnostic criteria for PMDD **36**
  biomedical experts' endorsement
    for 85–87
  concession to gynaecologists 136–137
  core symptoms included in **115**, 116
  discourse on shortcomings of 114–115
  and health insurance claims 139–140, 153
  minimum number of symptoms for
    diagnosis 86, 114
  typically mild changes included in 82–83
dysmenorrhea *see* period pain

E

education on menstrual physiology 3,
11–13, *12*, 142, 152–153, 156–157,
158–159
  call to action 160–164
  implications of gap in 24–25
  see also textbooks
embodied interpersonal stress,
Premenstrual Syndrome as 49–50
Emera, D. 14, 16, 18, 19, 134
emotional distress
  as biological in origin 40, 47, 51,
113–114
  as a cause of hysteria 27, 28, 30
  critical experts on 51, 66, 71, 76, 107
  cross-cultural reporting of 39
  and distressing experiences 32, 42, 47,
123, 162
  embodied interpersonal 49–50
  expert prioritisation of 64–67, 78–79,
80, 91, 103, 110, 150
  universal experience of 32, 123
  see also mood changes
epileptic seizures 113
exaggerating premenstrual problem *see*
premenstrual problems, exaggerating
extra-discursive analysis 58–59, **59**, 136

F

female body
  'for' having children 18, 19, 24, 161, 164
  as pathological. *see* 'femininity as debility'
myth informing 'the curse' discourse
'female body as mysterious' myth
  informing 'black box' discourse 19–20,
23, 124–144, *143*
  disciplinary dilemmas 136–141
    positivism vs social
constructionism 140–141
    psychiatry vs gynaecology 136–140
  ignorance of menstruation 124–130
    clinical interactions 128–130
    increasing distress around
symptoms 126–128
  reduction and mystification of menstrual
cycle 130–136, 152–153
    equating menstrual cycle with
'fluctuating hormones' only 131–133,
132, *134*, 135, 152–153
    mystification of contradictory
data 133–136, 142
  why this matters 144
'femininity as debility' myth informing 'the
curse' discourse 104–123, *122*
  blaming female sex hormones 104–108
  uptake of biomedical discourses by
others 107–108
  exaggerating premenstrual problem
114–120

estimating number of premenstrual
symptoms 116–118
estimating population prevalence
of 118–120, *119*, 121
gendered symptoms and treatments
110–114, **110**
PMS stereotype as perpetuated by
men 108–110, 120–121
why this matters 122–123
femininity, idealised 49
feminist psychology 51
feminists vs clinicians 140–141
fertility, myth of periods signalling 19
Figert, Anne 37–38, 51
First World War 32
Frank, Robert 32, **33**, 37
Freud, Sigmund 28, 31

G

gender myths
  co-creation of racial and 34
  descriptions of PMS influenced by
146–151, *148–149*, 152–153, 159–160,
180–181
  how and why participant descriptions of
PMS reflect key 145–155, *148–149*
  'hysterical/hormonal female' 4–5, 24,
63, 81, 106
  in media 37, *38*
  PMS stereotype as current incarnation
of 37, *38*, 40, *41*, 68
  LLPDD and 38
  unintended reproduction of 155, 156,
158, 159
  see also 'all in the mind' gender myth;
'female body as mysterious' myth
informing 'black box' discourse;
'femininity as debility' myth informing
'the curse' discourse
gender relations and advent of
capitalism 30–31
gender, science of 31
gendered and contested diagnosis of
Premenstrual Syndrome 37–42
gendered perspectives on Premenstrual
Syndrome 108–114, 120–121
  gendered symptoms 110–112, **110**, **111**
  gendered treatments 112–114
  PMS stereotype as perpetuated by
men 108–110
glossary x–xii
Gold, Ellen 21, **60**, 61
Grounded Theory Methods 57
Gunter, Jen 3
gynaecology vs psychiatry 136–140, 142

H

Halbreich, U. 40
health apps 188n102

health insurance 139–140, 153
healthcare professionals
    call to action 161–163
    see also clinicians
history of medicine, female health in
    26–29, 185n11
hormones
    blaming female sex 104–108
        uptake of biomedical discourses by
            others 107–108
    categorisation of sex 183–184n36
    cited as a causal factor in premenstrual
        symptoms 105, 106, 126
    discovery of sex 32
    equating menstrual cycle with
        'fluctuating hormones' only 131–133,
        132, *134*, 135, 152–153
    implication in mood disorders 187n68
    maintaining 'hormonal' discourse
        despite contradictory data
        133–136, 142
    move from hysterical to hormonal
        32–36, 40, 186n48
        why this matters 42–43
    reduction of menstrual psychology to 20,
        22–23
    in typical depiction of menstrual
        cycle *12*
Horney, Karen 1, 36–37
hypochondriasis 27, 28
hysterectomy 112–114, 129
hysteria
    association with *hypochondriasis* 27, 28
    female prevalent symptoms in history of
        medicine 26–29, 185n11
    first references to emotional
        symptoms 27
    from hysterical to hormonal
        emergence of biomedical PMS 26,
            32–36, 40, 186n48
        why this matters 42–43
    key political and philosophical influences
        on 29–32
    two types 26
'hysterical/hormonal female' myth 4–5,
    24, 63, 68, 81, 106
    in media 37, *38*
    PMS stereotype as current incarnation
        of 37, *38*, 40, *41*, 68

I

inflammation 133, 142, 144, 159
    hs- CRP levels 20
    menstrual cycle and 20–22
interdisciplinary dilemmas 136–141,
    142–143
    positivism vs social
        constructionism 140–141
    psychiatry vs gynaecology 136–140

interviews
    discursive device notation 55, 174–175
    participants 53–55, **54**, 190n61
    question list 55, 169–172
    transcription notation 55, 61, 173
iron- deficiency anaemia 22–23, 50, 90,
    132–133, **132**, 159
    treating 163
iron levels 185n74

J

Jacobi, Mary Putnam 1
Johnson-Robledo, I. 17

K

Kahun Gynaecological Papyrus 26–27

L

Late Luteal Phase Dysphoric Disorder
    (LLPDD) 35, 38
lesbian couples 50

M

Mallia, Catriona **60**, 61, 119, **147**
mammals, menstruation in other 14, *15*
Marvan, Maria 49
maternal deaths 16, 18, 22, 156
medicalisation of mild premenstrual
    changes 82–89, **83**
    comparing medicalised symptoms by
        participant group 87–89, **88**
    contradictory expert discourses
        85–87, 101
    contradictory patient discourses
        84–85, 101
    critical experts' opposition to 83–84
    reflected in PMS stereotype 82–83
men
    comparing non-sex-specific symptoms
        associated with PMS in women
        and 105–106, 107
    maintaining patriarchy 30–31, 40
    perpetuation of PMS stereotype
        108–110, 120–121
menopause
    as 'cure' for premenstrual symptoms 112
    health in 3, 4
    PMS stereotype applied to menopausal
        women 40, *41*
menstrual cycle, reduction and mystification
    of 11–25, 130–136, 152–153
    equating cycle with 'fluctuating
        hormones' only 131–133, **132**, *134*,
        135, 152–153
    experts' difficulty in distinguishing
        between healthy and debilitating
        premenstrual symptoms 130–131
    lack of knowledge about menstrual
        cycle 124–130, 141–142, 156–157

menstrual physiology beyond
hormones 20–23
blood loss and iron deficiency 22–23
inflammation 20–22
mystification of contradictory data
133–136, 142
reasons for menstruation 13–16
evidence base 14–16
myths 16–20, 183n28
teaching reduced version of menstrual
physiology 11–13, *12*
textbook omissions 11, 135–136, 142,
152–153, 159, 165–166
use of terms relating to healthy
premenstrual physiology 131–132, **132**
why this matters 23–25, 144
menstrual fluid 16–17, 125–126
Menstrual Matters website 6
menstrual/menopause leave 4
menstruation
dirty/toxic metaphors 125–126, **126**
evidence base for 14–16
ignorance over purpose of 124–126
myths 16–20, 183n28
periods clean out womb 16–17
periods help prepare for
pregnancy 17–18
periods signal fertility 19
we don't know why we have
periods 19–20
prevalence in mammals 14, *15*
metaphors
to describe premenstrual experiences,
top 10 **59**
dirty/toxic 125–126, **126**
methods *see* study comparing discourses
on Premenstrual Syndrome
mind over matter *see* premenstrual
changes, psychologisation of
minorities *see* racialised minorities
miscarriage 24–25, 164, 182ch1n8
mood changes 52
biomedical PMS described as only or
mainly negative 64–66, 78, 146, 150
concurrent in PMS patients and
partners 106
consulting a doctor about 90, 91–92, **92**
critical experts' positioning of 79
cultural differences in likelihood of
mentioning 39, 40, 48
differentiating normal from
problematic 130
experts' overemphasis of 87–88, **88**, 110
implicating of hormones in 187n68
in lists of most common premenstrual
symptoms 67, **67**
medicalisation of 101
physical symptoms positioned as 'less
debilitating' than 65–66, 91, 99, 101, 103

PMS stereotype and biomedical
positioning of 71–73
prioritised over pain 80, 90, 103, 146
severe 74, 78, 79, 80–81, 162
sex differences in causes of 105–106, 109
see also emotional distress
moral judgements 40
Mother Nature 40, *41*
Mukwende, Malone 5

N

neuroactive steroids 131
neurotransmitters 131
normal curve analogies 95–99, 102–103
notation
discursive device 55, 174–175
transcription 55, 61, 173

O

oestrogen 32, 36, 105
oophorectomy 112, 113, 129
Othering of women and racialised
minorities 17, 24, 30, 79, 81
ovulation 19, 110, 191–192n9

P

pain
cultural differences in pain beliefs 70
diminishing women's accounts of 63, 90,
93, 101, 103, 150, 162
mood changes prioritised over 80, 91,
103, 146
underemphasis of pain-related
experiences 93, **94**
see also period pain
participants, interview 53–55, 190n61
anonymisation 55
characteristics and information **54**
participant background survey 167–168
patients
comparisons of descriptions of PMS
symptoms in population data vs
145–146, **147**
consulting a doctor over premenstrual
symptoms 69–70, 90, 91–92, **92**, 128–
130, 141
descriptions of PMS 66–67, **67**, 79, 95
disbelief in (racialised) experiences of 24,
30, 42–43, 63, 68–70, *69*, 79, 81
estimating number of PMS
symptoms 117–118
estimating prevalence of PMS 84,
118–119, *119*, 120, 121
first learning about PMS 128
gender myths influencing discourse
150–151, 153, 181
gendered symptoms 111–112, **111**
lack of knowledge about
menstruation 124–128, 141, 156

increasing distress around
symptoms 126–127
lists of most common symptoms **67**,
115–116, **115**
medicalisation of premenstrual
changes 84–85, **88**, 101
minimisation of debilitating menstrual
symptoms 89–90, **94**
perspectives on PMDD 77–78, 79
poor patient experiences and health
outcomes 156
surgery to 'cure' severe cyclical
symptoms 113–114
use of terms relating to healthy
premenstrual physiology 132–133, **132**
on why premenstrual symptoms
occur 108, 126
patriarchy 30–31, 40
period pain **88**, 95, 99, **115**
consulting a doctor over 90, **92**
minimisation of 90, 93–95, **94**, 97, 101
prioritising of mood changes
over 91, 103
as secondary dysmenorrhea 97
period poverty 3–4
personal, why this matters
black box 144
the curse 123
from hysterical to hormonal 43
mind over matter 81
reduction and mystification of menstrual
cycle 24–25
snatch-22 103
what counts as premenstrual
symptoms 63
Perz, Janette 49, 51
positionality 5–6
positivism vs social constructionism
140–141, 142–143
pre-eclampsia 18, 19
pregnancy 16
myth of periods helping prepare
for 17–18
premenstrual changes as simultaneously
'normal' and debilitating 82–103
biomedical labelling of most
common 99, **100**
clinical specialism typically responsible for
most common 99, **100**
medicalisation of mild changes 82–89, **83**
comparing medicalised symptoms by
participant group 87–89, **88**
contradictory expert discourses
85–87, 101
contradictory patient discourses
84–85, 101
critical experts' opposition to 83–84
minimisation of debilitating
symptoms 89–93

comparing minimised symptoms by
participant group 93–95, **94**
contradictory expert discourses 90–93
contradictory patient discourses 89–90
'snatch-22' paradox 82, 89, 95–99, 101, *102*
different diagnoses for severe physical
premenstrual symptoms 99
normal curve analogies 95–99
why this matters 102–103
premenstrual changes, psychologisation
of 64–81, *80*
'all in the mind' 67–73, 79, *80*, 81,
180, 181
biomedical perspectives and PMS
stereotype 71–73
Black and ethnic minorities 70
critical perspectives and PMS
stereotype 71
disbelief in patient experiences 68–70,
69, 79, 81
expert prioritisation of emotional
distress 64–67
biomedical PMS 64–66, **67**, 78
critical PMS 66, **67**, 78–79
patient PMS 66–67, **67**, 79, 95
'most common' symptoms **67**
PMDD 73–78
biomedical positioning 74–75
critical perspective 76–77
patient perspectives 77–78, 79
why this matters 80–81
Premenstrual Dysphoric Disorder (PMDD)
concept of priming 48
confusing PMS with 65, 72–73, 73–74
drug trial 191n1
DSM V diagnostic criteria **36**
biomedical experts' endorsement
for 85–87
concession to gynaecologists 136–137
core symptoms included in **115**, 116
discourse on shortcomings of 114–115
and health insurance claims
139–140, 153
minimum number of symptoms for
diagnosis 86, 114
typically mild changes included
in 82–83
estimated prevalence 119, *119*
a highly contested and gendered
diagnosis 38–39
hormonal causal discourse 105, 106
link between trauma and diagnosis of 50
misdiagnosis of 129
normal curve analogies in differentiating
PMS and 95–96, 97, 103
patients diagnosed with 127, 129
positioning of 73–78
biomedical perspective 74–75, 76–77,
77–78, 79

critical perspective 76–77
    patient perspectives 77–78, 79
psychiatry vs gynaecology
    and concession-based definition
        136–137, 142
    and shared ownership of PMDD
        138–139, 154
'relationship strain' a factor in 49
suggestion that physical premenstrual
    changes caused by 73, 85
top 10 countries publishing studies
    (1945–2018) 38–39, **39**
premenstrual exacerbation (PME) 75,
    98–99, 116
    of depression and anxiety 77
    of psychosis/severe emotional distress 98
premenstrual problems,
    exaggerating 114–120
    estimating number of PMS
        symptoms 116–118
    estimating population prevalence of
        PMS 118–120
Premenstrual Syndrome (PMS)
    bad science 145–151
    biomedical 64–66, **67**, 78
    biopsychosocial factors in 48–51, 62
    comparing descriptions of symptoms
        in participant groups vs population
        data 145–146, **147**
    comparing male and female experiences
        of non-sex-specific symptoms associated
        with 105–106, 107
    confusing PMDD with 65, 72–73,
        73–74
    critical 66, **67**, 78–79
    cross-cultural studies of symptoms 39, 49
    'defence' 34, 37
    definitions 47, 114–116, 121
        critical experts not invited to meetings
            on 140–141
        'good clinical intentions' for 154–155
        interdisciplinary concession-based
            136–137, 142
        RCOG clinical guidelines 35–36
    discursive mechanisms and extra-
        discursive factors affecting descriptions
        of 151–153, **152**, 158–159
    demonstrated intentions 153, **154**
    emergence of biomedical 26, 32–36,
        40, 186n48
        why this matters 42–43
    emergence of critical perspectives on 36–42
        PMS as a highly contested and
            gendered diagnosis 37–42
    estimating number of symptoms
        116–118, 121
    estimating population prevalence of 47,
        86, 118–120, **119**, 121
    first learned about 128, 130

gender myths influencing descriptions
    of 146–151, *148–149*, 152–153,
    159–160, 180–181
gendered perspectives 108–114, 120–121
good intentions 151–155
highly contested and gendered
    diagnosis 37–42
implications of expert and patient
    descriptions of 155–160
moral judgements and diagnostic tools 40
patient 66–67, **67**, 79, 95
psychiatry vs gynaecology
    and concession-based definition
        136–137, 142
    and shared ownership of PMS 138, 154
    RCOG clinical guidelines 35–36
    research publications
        1950–2018 35, *35*
        top 10 countries (1945–2018) 38–39, **39**
    see also stereotype, Premenstrual
        Syndrome; study comparing discourses
        on Premenstrual Syndrome
Premenstrual Tension (PMT) 32–34, **33**
prevalence of PMS, estimating 47,
    118–120, *119*, 121
    biomedical expert estimates 86, 118,
        119–120, 121
    critical experts 118
    patient estimates 84, 118–119, 120, 121
progesterone 34, 104, 135
psychiatry 51
    vs gynaecology 136–140, 142
psychologisation of premenstrual
    changes *see* premenstrual changes,
    psychologisation of
purposive sampling 53

R

racial biases in medical training 5
racial myths, co-creation of gender and 34
racialised minorities
    disbelief in patient experiences 24, 30,
        42–43, 63, 68–70, *69*, 79, 81, 146
    Othering of 17, 24, 30, 79, 81
    poor patient experiences and health
        outcomes 156
    unconscious bias towards 161–162
'relationship strain' a factor in PMS 49–50
religious
    affiliations and use of dirty/toxic
        metaphors 126, **126**
    myths about menstruation 16–17, 59
research
    call to action on 160–161
    inadequate 158
    publications
        1950–2018 35, *35*
        top 10 countries (1945–2018) 38–39, **39**
    questions 52

Romans, Sarah **60**, 61, 74, **147**
Romero, R. 14
Royal College of Obstetricians and
　Gynaecologists (RCOG) 35–36
Ruble, Diane 48

S

sampling 53
science
　bad 145–151
　call to action 160–161
　why this matters to
　　black box 144
　　the curse 122
　　from hysterical to hormonal 42
　　mind over matter 80–81
　　reduction and mystification of
　　　menstrual cycle 23
　　snatch-22 102
　　what counts as premenstrual
　　　symptoms 62–63
self-immolation 98
self-objectification 49
shell shock 32
'snatch-22' paradox 82, 89, 95–99,
　101, *102*
　different diagnoses for severe physical
　　premenstrual symptoms 99
　normal curve analogies 95–99
　why this matters 102–103
social constructionism vs positivism
　140–141, 142–143
society
　call to action in 163–164
　why this matters to
　　black box 144
　　the curse 123
　　from hysterical to hormonal 43
　　mind over matter 81
　　reduction and mystification of
　　　menstrual cycle 24
　　snatch-22 103
　　what counts as premenstrual
　　　symptoms 63
Sowemimo, Anabel 5
Spironolactone 135
spontaneous decidualisation 14–15
Stepan, Nancy 31, 34
stereotype, Premenstrual Syndrome
　67–68, 82
　biomedical perspective and 71–73
　critical perspective and 71
　as current incarnation of 'hysterical/
　　hormonal female' myth 37, *38*, 40,
　　41, 68
　and disbelief in patient experiences
　　68–70, *69*, 79, 81
　medicalisation of menstrual cycle
　　reflected in 82–83

as perpetuated by men 108–110,
　120–121
study comparing discourses on
　Premenstrual Syndrome 52–61
　conducting Critical Realist Discourse
　　Analysis 55–61, 145, 158
　excerpts v. quotes and their
　　labelling 61
　step 1: Discursive Psychology
　　analysis 56
　step 2: (Rhetorical) Discourse
　　Analysis 56–58, 176–179
　step 3: Extra-discursive analysis 58–59,
　　59, 136
　step 4: Data triangulation 59–61, **60**
　interviews
　　discursive device notation 55,
　　　174–175
　　interview question list 55, 169–172
　　transcription notation 55, 61, 173
　participants 53–55, 190n61
　　anonymisation 55
　　background survey 167–168
　　characteristics and information **54**
　purposive sampling approach 53
　research questions 52
suffrage movement 31, 37
suicidal ideation 65, 76, 79, 86, 90, 93,
　97, 110
Sydenham, Thomas 27, 30, 31
symptoms, premenstrual
　blaming female sex (hormones)
　　for 104–108
　clinical interactions regarding 128–130
　comparing descriptions of symptoms
　　in participant groups vs population
　　data 145–146, **147**
　core symptoms **115**, 116
　cross-cultural studies 39, 49
　different diagnoses for severe physical 99
　differentiating normal from
　　problematic 130–131, 142
　discourse on why symptoms occur
　　104–108, 120
　estimating number of 116–118, 121
　and exaggeration of premenstrual
　　problem 114–120
　and female-prevalent symptoms in history
　　of medicine 26–29, 185n11
　gendered symptoms and treatments
　　110–114, **110**, **111**
　inadequate research into causes and
　　treatment of 158
　minimisation of debilitating 89–95, **94**
　most common mentions by participant
　　group **67**
　tracking 129, 162
　what counts as 47–63
　　biopsychosocial factors in PMS 48–51

study comparing discourses on 52–61
why this matters 62–63
see also abdominal pain; 'bloating';
emotional distress; mood changes;
premenstrual changes as simultaneously
'normal' and debilitating; premenstrual
changes, psychologisation of

T

tampon tax 4
'tearfulness' 110–111
textbooks 142, 163–164
call for action 163, 164
racial biases in 5
review of 11, 135–136, 152–153, 159,
165–166
transcription notation 55, 61, 173
transgender people 55
treatments for premenstrual symptoms
anti-inflammatory medications 22, 99, 135
first-line 20, 21

gendered 112–114
Spironolactone 135

U

unconscious bias 161–162
Ussher, Jane 40, 49, 51, **166**

V

Veith, I. 28

W

Wagner, G. 14
Warner, P. 50
water retention 111–112, 131–132, **132**
Willis, Thomas 1, 29–30
womb, 'wandering' 27, 29
Women's Health Across the Nation
project 20
women's health, moving forward
in 160, 164
workforce, women in 40